People Handling
Handbook

Allied Training
Unit 6C Kerlogue Business Park,
Kerlogue, Wexford.
M: 086 7778400
T: 053 91 40655 / 40654
W: www.alliedtraining.ie

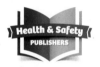

This handbook has been designed to be used in conjunction with training, but not on its own as a replacement for training.

This handbook gives guidance on the handling of people who require assistance; for information on the handling of loads refer to the booklet Manual Handling - course notes.

Grace Killeen

Introduction

Back pain is a very common occurrence (it is estimated that four out of five of all adults will experience back pain at some stage in their lives). Manual handling accounts for approximately 40% of all reported workplace injuries[2] and this has a serious impact on employers and Individual.[1] But the good news is that employers can take measures to reduce the likelihood of workplace injury and employees can reduce the chances of developing back pain by applying some basic measures to their lives, and, in particular, in the workplace.

In the healthcare sector this general problem of risk of injury from manual handling can take the particularly high risk form of the manual handling of people, in which a multitude of factors can affect the situation. It is important to remember that not only can the handler be harmed but also the individual being assisted can suffer bruising, injury, pain or discomfort as a consequence of inappropriate management of manual handling. It is also important to note that professional codes of conduct require prevention of abuse and that "Physical abuse is any physical contact which harms clients or is likely to cause them unnecessary and avoidable pain and distress. Examples include handling the client in a rough manner, poor application of manual handling techniques or unreasonable physical restraint. Physical abuse may cause psychological harm."[3]

The law requires manual handling training in the workplace, but the knowledge acquired there of correct technique and the factors affecting back health can be applied outside the workplace, and remembering these can have a significant impact on the well-being of individuals in their everyday lives. We know that back pain is most common in tasks that involve:

- Stooping, bending or poor sitting posture;
- Stretching, twisting and over-reaching;
- Prolonged periods in one position;
- Lifting heavy or bulky loads;
- Carrying, pushing or pulling loads awkwardly or over long distances;
- Repetitive activity;
- Working beyond the range of our normal abilities and/or stamina;
- Working when physically or mentally tired.

Prevention is better than cure and many of these factors in our work are within our control and by the adoption of different working practices can be eliminated or reduced so that risk of painful injury can also be eliminated or reduced. The causes of back pain are often innocuous and, from the medical evidence, the Royal College of General Practitioners and the Faculty of Occupational Medicine have derived the following three key messages to people on how to manage back pain:

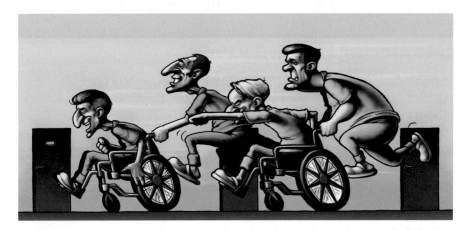

- ➡ Stay active;
- ➡ Try simple pain relief;
- ➡ If you need it, seek advice.

If you are suffering from back pain and suddenly notice any of the following symptoms visit a doctor straight away: [2]

- ➡ Difficulty passing or controlling urine;
- ➡ Numbness around your back passage or genitals;
- ➡ Numbness, pins and needles, or weakness in both legs;
- ➡ Unsteadiness on your feet.

The benefits of managing manual handling effectively are significant not only for employees and the organisations to which they belong, but also for anyone who needs assistance in accomplishing manual handling tasks. Training is an essential part of managing manual handling but it must be complemented by sound risk assessments, safe systems of work, good management processes, clear instructions, the suitable provision of equipment and a workplace culture and working attitudes that support it. When we undertake the manual handling of people, applying all these factors successfully will ensure that the individual concerned receives the highest standard of care and has his or her needs met appropriately.

Unit 1
Legislation

Introducing Health & Safety

Consider for a moment what might happen if a serious accident occurred in your organisation. How might it affect you, your colleagues, the person you are assisting or your organisation?

an accident occurs because of an organisations failure to manage risks, action might be taken leading to fines, imprisonment or both.

In addition an injured person might seek to be compensated for their injuries, as well as suffering and the loss of earning. The hidden costs of accidents in the workplace can quickly escalate.

There are three reasons to manage health and safety effectively:

MORAL It's not acceptable for workers, or the people they assist, to suffer injury and ill health as a result of doing their job.

LEGAL The law requires that organisations assess risk and where identified put in place measures to reduce risk to the lowest level so far as is reasonably practicable.

ECONOMIC In addition to fines and increased insurance premiums other factors such as loss of reputation and increased staff turnover can quickly add up.

The Irish Legal System

Irish Law consists of constitutional, statute and common law.

Constitutional law is the highest law in the state and provides the authority for all other law.

Statute law refers to acts of the Oireachtas for example the "Safety, Health and Welfare at Work Act 2005" while common law refers to the application of precedents previously set.

Health and Safety Legislation

Health and safety legislation in Ireland (for example The Safety, Health and Welfare at Work Act and its associated General Application Regulations) is designed to secure and improve the Safety, Health and Welfare of people at work by advocating a preventative "Risk Assessment" approach to managing safety.

The Health and Safety Authority (HSA) is the statutory body in Ireland responsible for the enforcement of occupational health and safety law and reports directly to the Minister for Jobs, Enterprise and Innovation.

Terminology

As health and safety jargon can often be difficult to understand a number of common phrases and statements are explained below.

Good practice represents what is generally expected by law or **Best practice** which may go beyond what is legally required.

Guidance is available in many different forms and available in publications. Guidance is not mandatory and therefore you do not have to follow it, however, it is based on considerable experience and is, therefore, often a good starting place for employers seeking ways to reduce risk.

Accident means an accident arising out of, or in the course of employment which, in the case of a person carrying out work, results in personal injury.

Hazard means a source or a situation with the potential for harm in terms of human injury or ill-health, damage to property, damage to the environment, or a combination of these.

Risk means the likelihood that a specified undesired event will occur due to the realisation of a hazard by, or during work activities, or by the products and services created by work activities. A risk always has two elements: the likelihood that a hazard may occur and the consequences of the hazardous event. Risk is also determined by the number of people exposed as well as how often.

Risk Assessment means the process of evaluating and ranking the risks to safety and health at work arising from the identification of hazards at the workplace. It involves estimating the magnitude of risk and deciding whether the risk is acceptable or whether more precautions need to be taken to prevent harm.

Reasonably Practicable means that an employer has exercised all due care by putting in place the necessary protective and preventive measures, having identified the hazards and assessed the risks to safety and health likely to result in accidents or injury to health at the place of work concerned and where the putting in place of any further measures is grossly disproportionate having regard to the unusual, unforeseeable and exceptional nature of any circumstance or occurrence that may result in an accident at work or injury to health at that place of work.

Dangerous Occurrence means an occurrence arising from work activities in a place of work that causes or results in:

- ⇥ the collapse, overturning, failure, explosion, bursting, electrical short circuit discharge or overload, or malfunction of any work equipment,
- ⇥ the collapse or partial collapse of any building or structure under construction or in use as a place of work,
- ⇥ the uncontrolled or accidental release, the escape or the ignition of any substance,
- ⇥ a fire involving any substance, or any unintentional ignition or explosion of explosives, as may be prescribed

Competent Person a person is deemed to be a competent person where, having regard to the task he or she is required to perform and taking account of the size or hazards (or both of them) of the undertaking or establishment in which he or she undertakes work, the person possesses sufficient **training, experience** and **knowledge** appropriate to the nature of the work to be undertaken.

The Safety, Health and Welfare at Work Act 2005

The Safety, Health and Welfare at Work Act 2005 applies to employers, employees in all employments and to the self-employed in the interests of securing a preventive approach to occupational health and safety. The 2005 act updates, repeals and replaces its predecessor, the Safety, Health and Welfare at Work Act 1989. The most relevant aspects are introduced below.

Duties of Employers

Section 8 of the Act requires every employer to ensure, so far as is reasonably practicable, the safety, health and welfare at work of all of his or her employees. The general duties of the employer set out in Section 8 broadly reflect in criminal legislation the common law principle of the duty of care. The duties cover:

- ⇥ The management and conduct of work activities

- ➡ The design, provision and maintenance of (I) safe workplaces (II) safe means of access to and egress from the workplace and (III) safe plant and machinery
- ➡ Providing safe systems of work
- ➡ Provision of adequate instruction, training and supervision and any necessary information
- ➡ Preparing risk assessments and safety statements as required by Sections 19 and 20 that take account of the general principles of prevention in Schedule 3 to the Act when implementing necessary safety, health and welfare measures
- ➡ Provision and maintenance of suitable personal protective equipment where risks cannot be eliminated, or where such equipment is prescribed
- ➡ To report accidents and dangerous occurrences to the Authority as may be required in Regulations under the Act
- ➡ To obtain, where necessary, the services of a competent person to assist in ensuring the safety, health and welfare of his or her employees

Duties of Employees

Section 13 is intended to protect the employee, fellow employees, and any other persons affected by the employee's actions. The employee has a duty under this section to co-operate with other duty holders so far as is necessary to enable those persons to comply with the appropriate relevant statutory provisions.

Section 13 provides for a range of duties on employees. An employee must:

- ➡ Comply with relevant laws and protect their own safety and health, as well as the safety and health of anyone who may be affected by their acts or omissions at work.
- ➡ Ensure that they are not under the influence of any intoxicant to the extent that they could be a danger to themselves or others while at work.
- ➡ Cooperate with their employer with regard to safety, health and welfare at work.
- ➡ Not engage in any improper conduct that could endanger their safety or health or that of anyone else.
- ➡ Participate in safety and health training offered by their employer.
- ➡ Make proper use of all machinery, tools, substances, etc. and of all personal protective equipment provided for use at work.
- ➡ Report any defects in the place of work, equipment, etc. which might endanger safety and health.

Safety Health and Welfare at Work (General Application) Regulations 2007 Chapter 4 of Part 2: Manual Handling of Loads

"manual handling of loads" means any transporting or supporting of a load by one or more employees and includes lifting, putting down, pushing, pulling, carrying or moving a load, which, by reason of its characteristics or of unfavourable ergonomic conditions, involves risk, particularly of back injury, to employees.

Duties of Employers

Employers are required to **AVOID** the need for employees to undertake any **hazardous** manual handling where there is a risk of their being injured. Regulations require the employer to organise the work to allow the use of mechanical or other means to avoid the need for the manual handling of loads by employees in the workplace.

Where moving and handling activities cannot be avoided employers must undertake a Risk Assessment of the activities. As a minimum this should consider the task, individual capability, the load and the working environment **(TILE)**.

Having assessed the level of risk employers must **REDUCE** the risk of injury to the lowest level so far as is reasonably practicable. Risk Assessments should be **RECORDED** and **REVIEWED** annually or whenever there is any reason to suspect they may no longer be valid or there has been a significant change in the manual handling activity to which it relates.

When assessing whether "Manual Handling of Loads" involve a risk of injury and in determining the steps necessary to reduce this the employer must consider the following:

- ➡ The physical suitability of the employee to carry out the activity (individual Risk Factors)
- ➡ The clothing, footwear or other personal effects being worn
- ➡ Their knowledge and training
- ➡ Whether they are in a group of employees identified as being especially at risk e.g Young workers, pregnant or returning to work from sickness.
- ➡ The results of any health surveillance

In addition employers should provide employees with general indicators such as the weight , stability of each load, the heaviest side and any other relevant information required for the safe moving and handing.

People Handling

Where an individual is the 'load' it is reasonable to assume that the assistance or 'manual handling' could be hazardous – people can be unpredictable, present with complex physical, mental and behavioural attributes, may be on medication or have medical issues. It would not, however, be reasonably practicable to say that people handling must be avoided at all cost e.g lifting legs into bed is hazardous but if someone needs that assistance in order to sleep in bed then it would not be considered 'reasonable' to say they must sleep in a chair in order to reduce the risk for the handler. This does not mean that the handler must be left to undertake this activity without suitable assessment, guidance and training.

There may well be instances when 'avoidance' is appropriate e.g. providing a profile bed to assist with sitting up in bed rather than a handler sitting them up.

It is required that a detailed Risk Assessment is undertaken of a persons individual needs and 'reasonable' interventions put in place that meet their needs but also take account of the handlers health and safety. This is seen as 'balanced-decision making'. In accordance with the 2010 "Guidance on Manual Handling Training System" Manual and Person Handling training programme attendees should:

➡ Have a basic knowledge of the legislation in relation to manual handling
➡ Acquire the basic knowledge of the functions of the back, how it can be injured and how to keep it healthy.
➡ Be able to carry out a personal/dynamic risk assessment for the task to be completed to determine if the load can be handled safely
➡ Be aware of the specific manual handling hazards identified in the task specific manual handling risk assessment and the measures to avoid or reduce the risk of injury including use of mechanical aids or reorganisation of the work activity
➡ Be able to state the main principles of safe manual handling and demonstrate practical application of the main principles of manual handling to relevant manual handling tasks in the workplace
➡ Be aware of the need to further develop manual handling skills in the workplace

Employees involved in patient/client handling in addition to the learning outcomes above should:

➡ Be aware of local policies and procedures related to handling patients which are relevant to their work area (such as bariatric guidelines, falls strategies, infection control, hoist management etc.)
➡ Be able to identify the additional factors which need to be included in a manual handling risk assessment when handling people
➡ Be aware of written documentation in relation to patient handling risk assessments in their work area

▣ Be aware of a range of handling aids available in their work area and the safe use of same

▣ Participate in a range of core patient handling techniques relevant to their work tasks

Safety Health and Welfare at Work (General Application) Regulations 2007 Chapter 2 of Part 2: Use of Work Equipment

The definition of work equipment, i.e. "any machinery, appliance, apparatus, tool or installation for use at work" in Regulation 2 is all inclusive. The most relevant aspects of these regulations are outlined below

Duties of Employers.

An employer shall ensure that:

Any work equipment provided for use by employees at a place of work complies, as appropriate, with the provisions of any relevant enactment implementing any relevant Directive of the European Communities relating to work equipment with respect to safety and health,

People Handling Considerations:
Equipment purchased must be fit for purpose taking account of the tasks, the work environment, the patient and employee needs. The provision of appropriate equipment has numerous benefits for the patient and the staff (e.g., the use of electric profiling beds to reduce high risk manual handling activities).

Effective equipment management will include:
▣ Identifying gaps in equipment needs;
▣ Being aware of the latest developments in equipment design;
▣ Ensuring the care and maintenance of equipment;
▣ Evaluation of equipment prior to procurement to ensure compatibility with existing furniture and equipment

Duties of Employees

As already identified under other legislation employees have a duty, when trained, to use equipment as instructed and ensure it is safe while using and when stored. All equipment should at every use be visually checked for damage, wear and tear, cleanliness and that it is the specific equipment required for that system of work i.e. designated on the individuals moving and handling plan.

Safety Health and Welfare at Work (General Application) Regulations 1993 Part X: Notification of Accidents and Dangerous Occurrence

Serious accidents in the workplace must be notified to the health and safety authority under the above Regulations.

→ Any death
→ Major injuries such as loss of sight or amputation
→ Injuries involving absence from work for more than three consecutive days not including the day of the accident
→ Dangerous occurrences such as the failing of lifting equipment
→ Reportable diseases

You can report accidents online by clicking on the "Report an Accident online" logo that appears on the Health and Safety Authority Home page www.hsa.ie or by completing the official IR1 form, The HSA only accept the pre-printed forms published by the Authority photocopies are not acceptable. Copies of the IR1 form are available from the Publications Section of the HSA by Telephoning 1890 289 389 or if calling from outside of the Republic of Ireland +353 1 6147000

Duties To The Person Being Assisted

As discussed earlier balanced-decision making is required when undertaking manual handling risk assessment of people. The risk assessment should take due account of any legislation which supports them as a vulnerable person.

Meeting the needs of the individual and their safety is as important as the health and safety of the carer.

The trainer of your course will highlight any specific legislation that is relevant regarding the individuals you care for, examples may include:

→ The Disability Act 2005
→ Mental Health Act 2001
→ Health and Social Care Professionals Act 2005
→ National Vetting Bureau (Children and Vulnerable Persons) Act 2012
→ Criminal Justice (Withholding of Information on Offences Against Children and Vulnerable Persons) Act 2012

Unit 2
The Musculoskeletal System

Our ability to move rests upon our use of the muscles and bones which constitute our musculoskeletal system. This system gives us our form and shape and provides our bodies with support and stability. It is responsible for bodily movements.

Constituents of the Musculoskeletal System	
Bones (skeleton)	Joints
Muscles	Ligaments
Tendons	Cartilage
Connective tissue (tissue that holds tissues & organs together)	Discs

The Skeleton

The skeleton is the body's supporting structure. The skeleton has the following important functions;

1. Support
The skeleton supports the body and maintains its shape.

2. Movement
The joints between bones allow for movement. The skeletal muscles are attached to the skeleton at a number of locations on the bones and they provide the power that enables movement.

3. Protection
The skeleton provides protection to a number of organs (e.g. the skull protects the brain and the ribcage protects the lungs and the heart).

Bones

The bones of the skeleton are divided into the:

➡ Appendicular skeleton (arm & leg bones);
➡ Axial skeleton (skull, spine, ribcage).

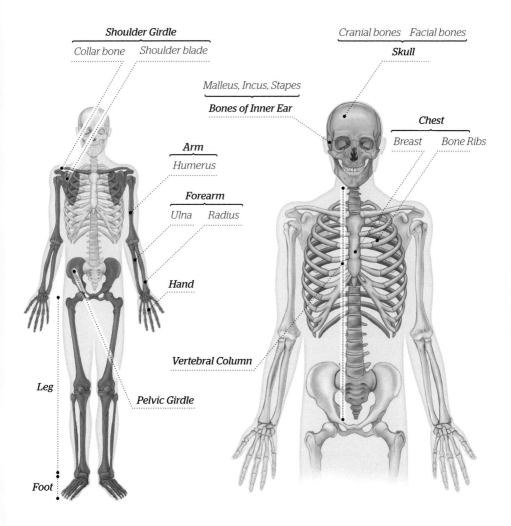

Fig. 1. Appendicular Skeleton

Fig. 2. Axial Skeleton

The human body consists of 206 hard, strong and minimally flexible bones of various sizes and shapes (some are long and some short; others are sesamoid, irregular or flat). In fact there are five types of bone in the human body each located differently

Type of Bone	Location
Long	Bones of the Limbs
Short	Wrist, Ankle
Flat	Bones of the Skull
Irregular	Spine, Hip
Sesamoid	Knee Cap

Long bones act as levers, flat bones protect organs and irregular bones protect organs and provide the origin for muscles.

Injury to bones

Fractures

A fracture is any break in the continuity of the bone. A fracture can result from forceful impact/stress or from a medical condition that causes the bones to weaken such as osteoporosis or cancer. Spinal fractures may pinch, compress or tear the spinal cord.

The Joints

The point at which two or more bones connect is known as a joint.
Joints are classified according to their structure and function:

Structure of Joint	Characteristics / Functions	Location
Fibrous	Joined by fibrous connective tissue; allows little or no mobility	Skull
Cartilaginous	Joined by cartilage; allows slight mobility	Vertebrae
Synovial	Not directly joined; allows a range of movement	Shoulder, Hip, Elbow, Knee.

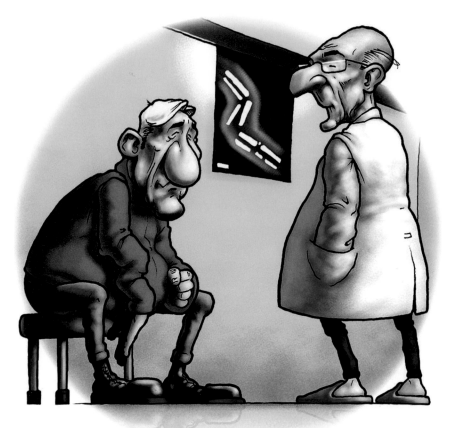

A bad break!!

Vertebral Facet Joints

Facet joints are joints of the spine. They connect each vertebra with the vertebrae above and below. These join and permit movement of the vertebral column.

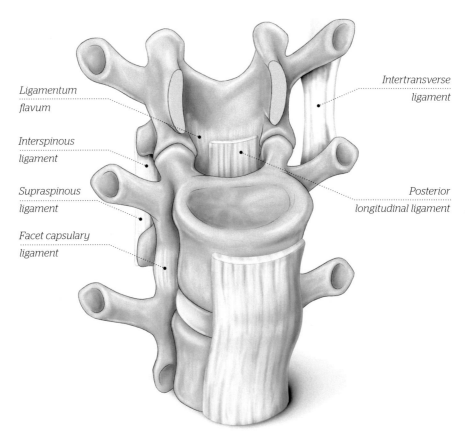

Ligamentum flavum

Interspinous ligament

Supraspinous ligament

Facet capsulary ligament

Intertransverse ligament

Posterior longitudinal ligament

Fig. 3. Facet Joint

Injury to Joints

Manual handling involving excessive bending, twisting and overextension may cause damage to the joints. Repeated lifting to and from a height may cause the facet joints to be pressed together creating intolerable strain. Over time this excessive strain may cause the joints to degenerate.

Muscles

Muscles are formed by the binding together of small muscle fibres into bundles (see figure 4). Muscles are classified as skeletal, cardiac or smooth.

Type of Muscle	Characteristics / Functions
Skeletal or voluntary muscle	Held by tendons to the bone; cause movement and maintain posture
Smooth or involuntary muscle	Located in the walls of the stomach, intestines, bladder, urethra, uterus, blood vessels and bronchi. These muscles are not under our conscious control
Cardiac muscle	Located only in the heart. This muscle is also involuntary

Muscles receive signals from the brain via nerves. Nerve impulses cause contraction of the muscle fibres. The contraction of muscle fibres causes the shortening of the muscle and causes movement at the joint.

The back muscles provide the power for movement in the spine (see figure 5). A group of muscles called the erector spinae muscles are active in the bending movement to the side and in the rotation of the spine. By flexing the spine, the external oblique abdominal muscles also play a part in spine movement. The latissimus dorsi muscle permits bending forward movement, and allows movement of the shoulder, head and arm. The quadriceps (thigh) muscles are also involved when lifting.

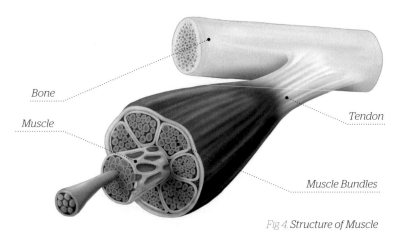

Bone

Muscle

Tendon

Muscle Bundles

Fig 4. Structure of Muscle

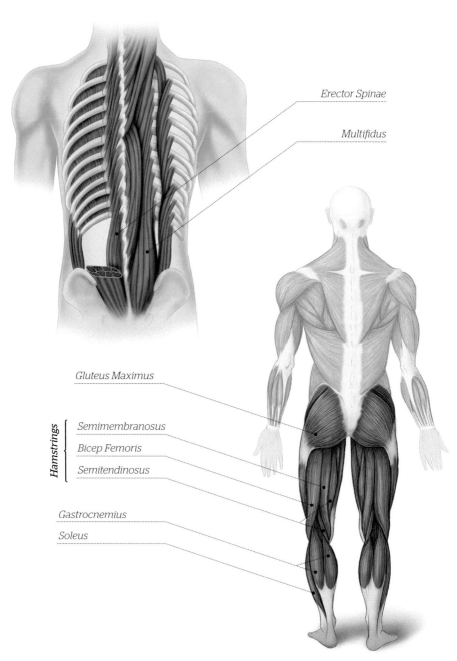

Erector Spinae

Multifidus

Gluteus Maximus

Hamstrings
Semimembranosus

Bicep Femoris

Semitendinosus

Gastrocnemius

Soleus

Fig 5. Muscles (Back)

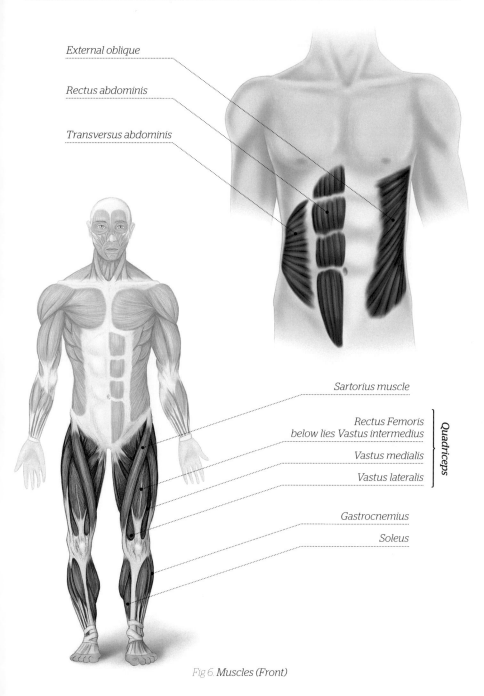

External oblique

Rectus abdominis

Transversus abdominis

Sartorius muscle

Rectus Femoris
below lies Vastus intermedius

Vastus medialis

Vastus lateralis

Quadriceps

Gastrocnemius

Soleus

Fig 6. Muscles (Front)

Injury to Muscles

Muscles can be injured in a number of ways:

Movement	Example
Sudden, sharp or strong movement	Action when attempting to push a car
Repetitive low force contractions	Working at a production line
Prolonged static muscle work	Sitting for long periods of time
Awkward angle of pull of the muscle	Bending and twisting
Sudden increase of work intensity and/or workload	Soccer player may cause injury to hamstring when accelerating suddenly during a game

Ligaments

Ligaments connect bones to bones to form a joint. Cruciate ligaments are those that are crossed in pairs (i.e. they are arranged in an ‚x' form). Such ligaments can be found in the knee. This formation of ligament provides stability to the joint and permits a huge range of motion.

The posterior longitudinal ligament is found within the vertebral canal and it restricts the range of forward flexion or bending of the spine. The anterior longitudinal ligament is found on the anterior surface of the spine.

Injury to Ligaments

Ligaments in the back may become strained from incorrect lifting, bending and twisting movements. It is these movements that may put our backs under constant or repeated strain. When ligaments become over-stretched they may lose their ability to hold the joints of the back in their correct position resulting in back sprain.

Tendons

Tendons are composed of fibrous connective tissue that connects muscle to bone (e.g. the Achilles tendon located behind the ankle, which is the thickest and strongest tendon in the human body).

Cartilage

Cartilage is composed of flexible connective tissue. It is found at the joints between bones, ear, nose, bronchial tubes and the intervertebral discs. Fibrocartilage is present in the annulus (see figure 7) of the intervertebral discs.

Connective Tissue

Connective tissue holds tissues and organs together.

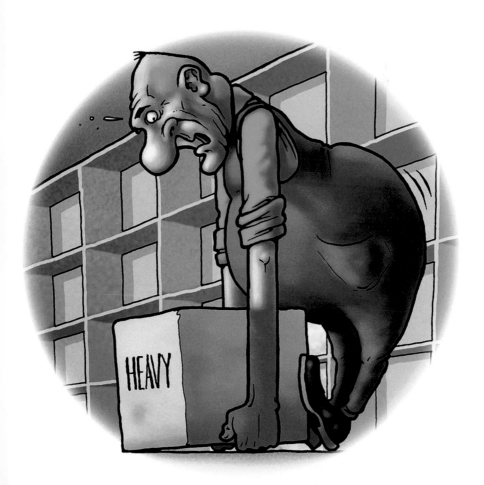

Unit 3
Intervertebral Disc

Discs are located between the vertebrae. Each disc has two functions: it forms a fibrocartilaginous joint which permits slight movement of the vertebrae and it works like a ligament by holding the vertebrae together.

The discs are composed of an outer part called the annulus, which surrounds the inner part, called the nucleus. The nucleus contains a gel substance with the consistency of a jelly (see fig.7). It is the nucleus of the disc that acts as the body's shock absorber between the vertebral bodies (see fig.8&9).

This jelly or nucleus may be forced out of the disc completely (herniated disc), causing pain as it exerts pressure on the nerve lying near the disc (see disc disorders).

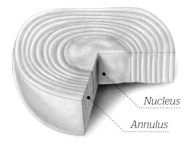

Nucleus

Annulus

Fig 7 Disc or Intervertebral Disc

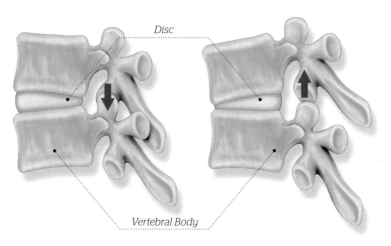

Disc

Vertebral Body

Fig 8 Movement of facet joints – bending backwards movement or extension

Fig 9 Movement of facet joints – bending forwards movement or flexion

Functions of the Disc

- ▷ Resists compression and shearing stresses on the spine;
- ▷ Acts as shock absorber;
- ▷ Separates vertebrae.

Because the discs have little in the way of direct blood supply they rely on a supply of nutrients through the blood vessels and tissues. Without an adequate supply of nutrients, the cells of the nucleus will die.

Injury to Discs

The purpose of figure 10 is to show a normal disc, moving down along the vertebral column you will see the various injuries that can occur and how it presents itself.

At the top of figure 10 you can see at a **normal disc** (a). A **normal disc** is perfectly formed and cushions the vertebrae above and below it. The **degenerative disc** (b) shown in figure 10 illustrates the natural process of degeneration of the disc as we age. The **degenerative disc** loses its flexibility, elasticity and ability to absorb shock. Next is shown the **bulging disc** (c), which may result when the disc moves out of its normal position. This may occur as part of ageing. It is more likely to occur gradually than suddenly. The **herniated disc** (d) shown next is similar to the bulging disc, but may result from a sudden injury sustained when lifting without bending the knees and keeping the back straight (i.e. bending at the waist). The **thinning disc** (e) shown may be indicative of degenerative disc disease. It is clear to see that the bony vertebrae on either side of the disc will rub together. The friction of the two

vertebrae may encourage the growth of the type of bone spurs (osteophytes) shown at the last level of figure 10 (**disc degeneration with osteophyte formation** (g)). By encroaching on the nerves these bony overgrowths may cause pain.

The abovementioned spinal injuries may occur as a result of repeated bending, twisting and lifting or sudden unexpected movements as well as the holding of awkward and/or static postures for long periods of time.

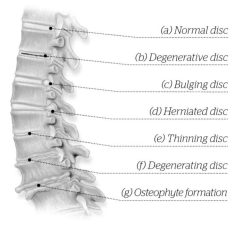

(a) Normal disc

(b) Degenerative disc

(c) Bulging disc

(d) Herniated disc

(e) Thinning disc

(f) Degenerating disc

(g) Osteophyte formation

Fig 10   Various disc injuries

Unit 4
Anatomy, Structure and Function of the Spine

Vertebral/Spinal Column

The vertebral column consists of 33 vertebrae separated by intervertebral discs. It serves to protect the spinal cord within the spinal canal.

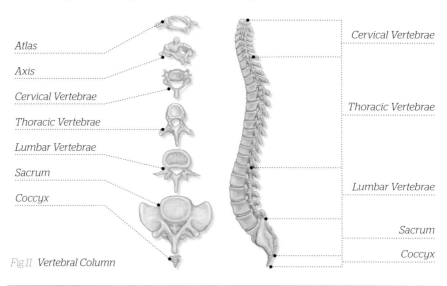

Atlas

Axis

Cervical Vertebrae

Thoracic Vertebrae

Lumbar Vertebrae

Sacrum

Coccyx

Cervical Vertebrae

Thoracic Vertebrae

Lumbar Vertebrae

Sacrum

Coccyx

Fig.11 Vertebral Column

Type of Vertebrae	No. of Vertebrae
Cervical	7 (C1-C7)
Thoracic	12 (T1-T12)
Lumbar	5 (L1-L5)
Sacral	5 (S1-S5) Fused
Coccygeal	4 Fused-Tail Bone

Each vertebra is composed of a front segment (vertebral body) and a back segment (vertebral neural arch) (see fig.12).

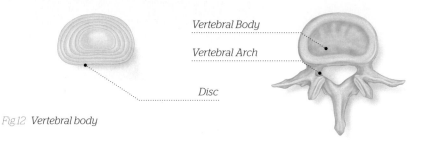

Vertebral Body

Vertebral Arch

Disc

Fig 12 Vertebral body

Functions of the Vertebral/Spinal Column

Function	Description
Protection	Protects the spinal cord, which it encloses
Movement (see figure 13 below)	Permits movement of the trunk: forward, backward, and left and right bending
Support	Supports the head
Production	Produces red blood cells
Attachment	Provides structural attachment for the ribs

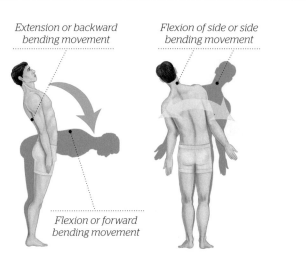

Extension or backward bending movement

Flexion of side or side bending movement

Rotation or twisting/turning

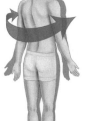

Flexion or forward bending movement

Fig 13 Movement of the Trunk

Unit 5
Posture & Back Pain

Posture

Learning and maintaining good posture is a sure method to prevent back pain. Remember the spine is not naturally straight: it has natural curves both slightly forward (in the lumbar region) and backward (in the thoracic region). A neutral or good posture is ensured when the ears, shoulders, hips, knees and ankles are aligned, whether sitting or standing. To achieve this, imagine a plumb line running from your ears down through your upper body to your legs and your feet (see figure 14 on the right).

Back Pain

Back pain may occur as a consequence of excessive wear and tear, incorrect posture, incorrect lifting techniques, prolonged heavy physical work, being overweight, lack of fitness, or underlying medical condition.

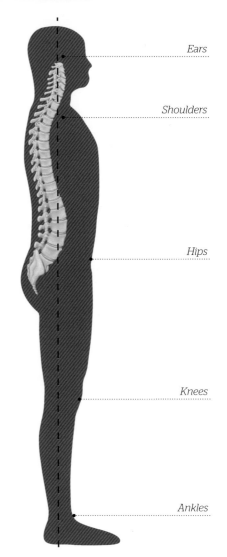

Ears

Shoulders

Hips

Knees

Ankles

Fig.14 Neutral or Good Posture

Types of Back Pain

Mechanical problems

▶ Herniated disc;
▶ Bulging disc.

Cause
Weakness or tear in the outer ring of the disc: the nucleus moves outside and soaks up copious amounts of water. The nucleus then swells rapidly making it impossible for it to move back into the disc.

Effect
The herniated disc may exert pressure on the nerves resulting in pain, numbness, and a reduction of strength and the ability to move.

Arthritis of facet joint

The facet joints are covered by smooth cartilage and surrounded by ligaments, and they are lubricated with a fluid called Synovial fluid. The facet joints may develop arthritis and become painful.

Cause
The affected facet joints develop bone spurs (a bony growth formed on normal bone). These bone spurs will restrict the space available for the nerve roots as they leave the spinal canal. Therefore the nerve roots become pinched causing pain, numbness and weakness.

Effect
Arthritis of the facet joints may cause back pain that worsens with twisting or bending backward movements.

Strained Muscles

Cause
Muscles fibres may become strained or abnormally stretched or torn as a consequence of overloading or sudden movement.

Internal problems

Back pain may also be caused by presence of an underlying medical condition.

Unit 6
Fitness & Flexibility

There are 4 elements to fitness:

➡ Endurance;

➡ Flexibility;

➡ Strength;

➡ Aerobic fitness.

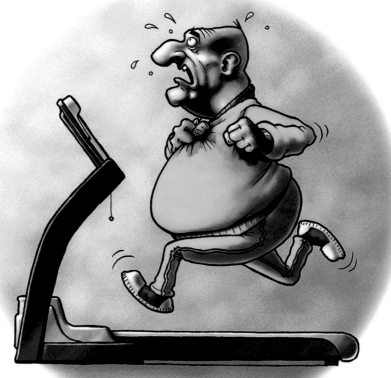

Talk to a Personal Trainer or your G.P. before you start exercising!!!

Endurance is the ability of the body to exert itself for a period of time. You can build up your endurance gradually (e.g. if you want to start jogging, begin with 10/13 minutes, and build slowly to 20 minutes). Experts recommend that those with average levels of fitness undertake at least 30 minutes per day of endurance activities such as walking, cycling, swimming, etc. Regular endurance activities not only improve posture and balance but also promote better health and weight control.

Flexibility refers to the ability of your joints and muscles to move within a certain range. The degree of flexibility varies from one person to another. Flexibility of joints can be increased by exercise and stretching. Stretching may be done after endurance and strength activities. Experts advise holding your stretch for 10/15 seconds without bouncing. Stretching incorrectly may cause harm.

Strength of muscle assists the protection of joints and muscles from injury (e.g. the abdominal and back muscles support the back during lifting). Muscle strength can be increased through special weight/strength training programmes. Strong muscles improve mobility and posture.

Aerobic fitness improves the function of the heart; it also improves the function of the lungs as it increases circulation efficiency and reduces blood pressure.

> **REMEMBER!**
> Before undertaking any stretching, strengthening or training programme always seek the advice of your G.P. and seek the professional advice of a personal trainer or your local fitness centre/gym instructor.

Unit 7

Ergonomics

Ergonomics is the application of scientific information concerning human beings to the design of objects, systems of work and environments for human use. Ergonomics should be an integral part of effective risk control. In healthcare settings, ergonomics is the matching of the carer to the task and an effective match will help to ensure:

- Work efficiency;
- Health and safety;
- Comfort, ease of use and enablement.

Key aspects in healthcare settings include:

Clear communication: verbal, non-verbal and written communication should ensure all involved in the activity have a full understanding of what is going to happen.

Sufficient space: every activity should have an optimum space to ensure the activity can be accomplished easily and efficiently.

Slip and trip hazards: planning and preparation (dynamic risk assessment) reduce the likelihood of unrecognised or unmanaged risks.

Appropriate equipment: should have been assessed as suitable for the individual, fit for the purpose, being used by a trained carer and clean and safe for use. If this is done the likelihood of accidents will be reduced.

Height adjustable work surfaces: reduce postural strain during work activities by using equipment such as a height adjustable bed to deliver personal care.

Training and supervision: appropriate and sufficient training will enable carers to work more safely and efficiently. Adequate supervision is necessary to support carers in achieving the standard required and enabling them to apply their training in the workplace.

Unit 8
Risk Assessment

There are two levels of risk assessment:

1. The formal, written risk assessment required by legislation, which should be carried out by a competent person.
2. The personal assessment of risk (dynamic risk assessment), which should be done by every individual before they undertake a task – this is the 'Stop, Think before you Do' level of assessment which people do in everyday life for ordinary tasks such as crossing the road.

1. Formal risk assessment

The process of risk assessment is straightforward and should:

1. Identify the hazard.
2. Decide who could be harmed and how.
3. Evaluate the risk.
4. Devise a plan aimed at eliminating or reducing the risk.
5. Put the plan in action and review.

Risk assessment will identify whether or not there are workplace manual handling activities and if these activities are 'hazardous'. Where risk assessment identifies a manual handling hazard, we are require to:

- ▶ Avoid the hazardous handling as far as is reasonably practicable;
- ▶ Assess hazardous handling that cannot be avoided;
- ▶ Reduce the risks to the lowest level reasonably practicable; and
- ▶ Review the assessment if the circumstances change.

Where the handling activity consists of assisting an individual to move or be transferred, the risks are self-evident and would often be considered hazardous.

Avoidance

Where it is reasonably practicable to avoid the hazardous handling then this approach should be considered. This is not necessarily avoidance of the task but maybe rather avoidance of the hazardous element of the task. It does not mean the individual should not be moved or assisted, but it does mean that a balanced decision must be made:

> *"A balanced decision is one that takes account of all relevant factors, balances the requirements of all legislation and the needs of the people involved. It aims to find a workable solution, rather than one party dictating an outcome to another"* [6]

Examples of 'avoidance' are:

- Using a profile bed to bring an individual into a sitting position (see Fig. 15)
- Lifting an individual with a hoist and sling (see Fig. 16)
- Turning and supporting an individual inside or lying on the bed with an in-bed turning device and hoist (see Fig. 17)
- Lifting legs into the bed using a mechanical leg-lifter.

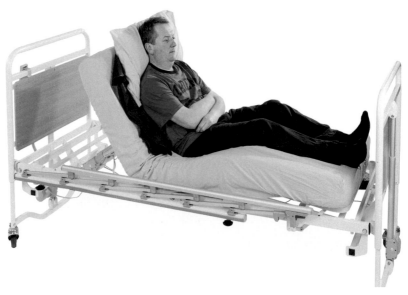

Fig 15

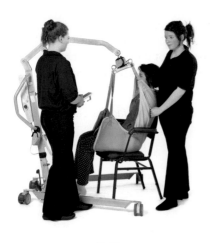

Fig.16

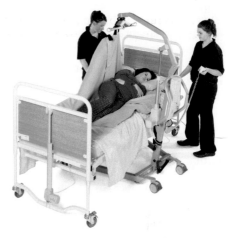

Fig.17

Assessment

The main elements of a manual handling risk assessment are commonly analysed using the framework TILEO:

T – task
I – individual capability of the person doing the task
L – load (individual or object) to be moved
E – environment where the task is being executed and equipment required
O – any other factor

A task analysis will gather information and then all the factors must be considered.

Where the 'load' is an individual, a considerable amount of information about that individual will be needed in order to understand his or her needs and abilities and to ensure that a suitable handling intervention is used.

A written assessment of the individual's needs should consider aspects such as the following:

- Physical ability and level of independence;
- Behaviour (predictability and compliance);
- Ability to communicate and level of cognition;
- Weight, height and body shape;
- Vision and hearing;
- Levels of pain and/or medication;
- Tissue viability (vulnerability to bruising, shearing, friction, pressure, etc);
- Infection control requirements
  (use of protective equipment such as aprons or gloves);
- History of falls;
- Comfort needs;
- The individual's expectations, wishes and concerns (including any religious, cultural and social issues);
- How much help the individual will require;
- Handling constraints (e.g., catheters, wound dressings, medical condition, etc).

Risk reduction

Establishing a suitable system of work with clear instruction on how it should be implemented should reduce the risks to a 'reasonable' level. For the moving and handling of people, such a system of work will be an individual 'handling plan' and this should describe the transfers required, the number of people needed to assist, the equipment to be used and any other information necessary. This handling plan should be:

- Sufficiently detailed (e.g., number of people required, sling size, type of attachment and attachment points to be used);
- Accessible to all those who need to read it;
- Read and complied with by those undertaking the activity;
- Reviewed regularly and, in particular, if there are changes in the circumstances, or if there has been an accident/incident.

Generic assessments and written protocols can save time and reduce duplication of documentation for tasks that are repeated such as the use of a hoist.
A generic assessment and/or protocol should:

- Identify the risks associated with the task (e.g., using a hoist or a sling);
- Give instruction on how to carry out the task (e.g. how to use a hoist or apply a sling).

Protocols should form the basis of a training programme. If a hoist or sling is used for an individual, generic information about using it should be available for reference alongside the individual's specific handling plan. Any differences or additional points relevant to the specific individual must be identified on his or her handling plan (e.g., which type or size of sling and which points of attachment are be used).

2. Dynamic (Personal) Risk Assessment

The individual's moving and handling plan must be followed as it is the instruction on how to assist him or her. If there is any reason to suspect that it no longer applies then this should be reported and the assessment reviewed. However, people pose challenges that are different from inanimate loads such as boxes. Their mood may change, they become tired, they do not want to do something and they can change their minds. This adds an additional dimension to the risks involved in the manual handling of people and it must be taken into account. For this reason, before assisting an individual, an 'on the spot' assessment should be made in order to check that the written system of work remains likely to apply.

It is beneficial to use the headings in the TILE or TILEO acronym as the basis for this dynamic assessment. For example:

T - Task

▶ What is the task (e.g., supporting for personal care in bed or a standing transfer?)
▶ How far must the individual be transferred?
▶ How often does the task need to be repeated?
▶ Is there risk of sudden unexpected movement?
▶ How long is the task going to take?
▶ Is it repetitive?

I - Individual Capability

▶ Is this task within my physical capability?
▶ Do I need help?
▶ Have I sufficient knowledge, training and skill?
▶ Does this task require unusual strength or height?
▶ Does this task pose a risk to people who are pregnant or have health issues?
▶ Am I wearing the correct footwear, clothing or protective items?
▶ Have I taken into account the need to manage cross-infection?

L - Load (An Individual)

➡ Have I read the specific handling plan?
➡ Can the individual communicate with me?
➡ How much can she or he do for herself or himself?
➡ Is the individual co-operative?
➡ Is the individual's behaviour predictable?
➡ How much help does the individual need?
➡ Does the individual have special needs owing to skin or tissue fragility?
➡ Is the individual in pain or discomfort and does the individual require medication?
➡ Does the individual have a history of falls?

E - Environment and Equipment

➡ Is there sufficient space?
➡ Is the area clear?
➡ What is the flooring like?
➡ What height is the working surface?
➡ Is the lighting or ventilation going to affect the task?
➡ Have I the right equipment?
➡ Am I trained in how to use the equipment?
➡ Have I checked the equipment for safety and cleanness?

O - Other Factors

➡ Does the task require specialist knowledge or information (e.g., dementia training)?
➡ Are there issues of mental capacity?
➡ Is the individual expressing concerns about being assisted?

Unit 9
Manual Handling of People

We must be clear from the outset that the manual handling of people is not just a health and safety issue but is also the meeting of a care need.

Manual handling is any transporting or supporting of a load, and includes lifting, lowering, pushing, pulling, carrying or moving by hand or bodily force.

Supporting activities using static postures are commonly seen in healthcare work (e.g. supporting limbs, holding an individual in a side lying position for personal care, washing, dressing, administering medication and many more). These supporting activities are likely to cause postural strain, with the potential for resulting injury, and must be risk assessed in the same way as the activities used to assist an individual to move.

Meeting mobility needs

Manual handling of people, as a load is undertaken when they cannot move without assistance. It is about meeting their mobility needs and in healthcare we prefer to describe this as 'moving and handling'.

The degree of assistance a person requires will depend on the activity level of the individual and a higher level of assistance generally increases the risks to the handler. The handling of people is recognised as hazardous for a range of reasons and the approach below should be applied for both static work and assisting mobility:

- ◗ Avoid hazardous handling as far as is reasonably practicable;
- ◗ Assess what cannot be avoided;
- ◗ Reduce the risk of injury to the lowest level reasonably practicable;
- ◗ Review and record.

Note that 'avoid' does not mean an individual's needs are not met: our aim is to avoid any hazardous manual handling while still completing the task (e.g. a profile bed can be used to assist an individual to sit up in bed rather than two carers manually assisting him or her). Even in higher-risk situations a balanced decision must be made that ensures risks are managed at a reasonable level whilst the individuals needs are also met reasonably as well. What is to be considered 'reasonable' should be identified by a risk assessment made by a competent assessor.

The manual, 'full body' lifts undertaken in the past are now seen as high risk and as unacceptable or controversial and should and can generally be avoided in most healthcare settings.

An individual's activity or mobility needs can be categorised as follows:

Independent :
a) Complete – can move themselves without intervention.
b) Moderate – can move themselves but may use an aid or need extra time.

Dependent:
c) Supervision – needs verbal prompting or someone to setup aids.
d) Minimal assistance – contributes at least three quarters of the effort but light assistance is needed.
e) Moderate assistance – contributes at least half the effort and needs more assistance.

Completely Dependent:
f) Maximum assistance – contributes less than half the effort and needs significant assistance.
g) Total assistance – contributes less than a quarter of the effort if any, needs total assistance.

Type of assistance

The assistance required should be identified by risk assessment of the individual and this should be recorded in a handling plan to ensure consistency of management.

The aim of assistance

Our aim is to give the least level of assistance necessary for the individual to complete the desired movement. In practice this will involve the following considerations:

- Promote and maintain independent function wherever possible;
- If assistance is required, encourage the individual to do as much as he or she can independently and only with additional aids or physical intervention if necessary;
- If total assistance is required, make a careful risk assessment to identify the right equipment and the right number of handlers to complete the activity with a reasonable level of risk and effort.

Unit 10
Controversial techniques

Current guidance on practice[6] teaches us that some techniques for the manual handling of people which were used in the past would now be considered high risk and potentially harmful to either the carer or the individual or both. It is, therefore, unacceptable to use these techniques as a standard practice when assisting individuals to move.

The trainer delivering your course will give you information on these controversial techniques but the following list enumerates some of them and gives basic definitions of them:

A. Manual lifting all or most of an individual's body weight. (This may still be undertaken in exceptional circumstances as long as a specific and detailed risk assessment has been completed (e.g., by the emergency services). The law requires that hazardous handling should be avoided where possible and, where it cannot be avoided, a detailed risk assessment must be done.) Such lifts include:

- ➡ Top and tail lift;
- ➡ Orthodox or cradle lift;
- ➡ Through-arm or hammock lift;
- ➡ Australian or shoulder lift;
- ➡ Drag lift.

B. Drag lift or under-arm hook to assist an individual to stand, walk, move up the bed or sit forward in a chair or bed.

C. Bear-hug stand or pivot transfer to assist an individual to stand or move from seat to seat.

D. Pulling up by holding hands to assist an individual stand up from a chair or the floor. (N.B. this is not the same as holding hands and prompting an individual to stand as described later for an individual with dementia.)

Unit 11
Standard preparation

Preparation for Assistance[6]

The following lists give the standard preparation that should be undertaken before any type of assistance is given. It applies to all the methods described in the chapter on Methods of Assistance (additional specific preparation for a method is covered in that chapter).

Always:

- Read the individual's handling plan;
- Do a dynamic risk assessment to identify any additional factors which could affect the situation (e.g., create adequate space, consider the question, is anything likely to cause a distraction during the activity);
- Consider the optimum starting position for the individual and the handler;
- Identify the best form of communication for the individual (e.g., verbal, visual etc);
- If in doubt how to proceed then ask.

Prepare the environment and the equipment:

- Create sufficient space for the activity and clear any obstruction (e.g., as wires).
- Check that any routes to be used are clear and the destination point is ready;
- Consider any risks created by the environment and manage them;
- If transferring an individual, bring the departing and receiving points as close as possible;
- Collect the equipment assessed/prescribed for the individual and the activity;
- Check the equipment is clean, safe and ready for use (see fig. 18)
- Use the equipment in accordance with your training and the manufacturer's instructions;
- Report any equipment that is unsuitable or unsafe to use;
- Apply brakes where appropriate (see fig. 19)
- Adjust working height where appropriate, particularly height adjustable beds.

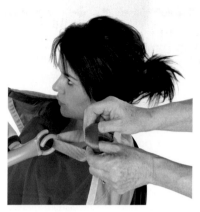

Fig 18

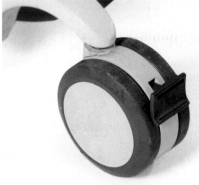

Fig 19

➡ If bed safe-sides are in situ, ensure these are lowered on the side you are working on to avoid reaching over and stooping;

➡ If kneeling, consider using a kneeling pad to protect your knees.

Prepare the individual:

➡ Explain the process and seek the individual's consent for the activity;

➡ Check the individual's current ability matches his or her assessed ability (physical, behavioural and cognitive);

➡ Check that the individual has no pain or discomfort, especially at any point where you will have direct contact with his or her body (e.g. hips, knees etc);

➡ Check that there is no additional action required (e.g. pain medication);

➡ Ensure the individual is wearing appropriate footwear and if they use spectacles or hearing aids that these are fitted;

➡ Check that the individual is in the optimum start position;

➡ Give clear instruction about the activity;

➡ Encourage the individual to participate as fully as his or her ability allows (see fig. 20)

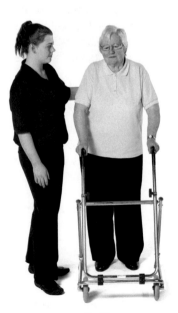

Fig.20

Prepare yourself:

➡ Ensure the activity is within your capability (e.g., physical, experience, skills);
➡ Use the appropriate number of people to assist;
➡ Apply your knowledge of biomechanical principles and the type of manoeuvre;
➡ Eliminate or reduce the need for any unnecessary movement (e.g., stooping, twisting, repetitious movements);
➡ Use the appropriate hold and method described for the activity;
➡ Adopt the basic walk stance, half- kneel stance or power squat depending on the activity.

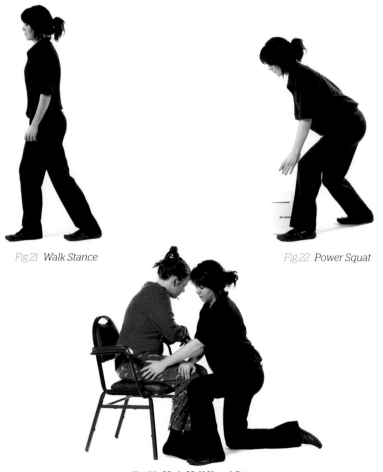

Fig.21 Walk Stance   *Fig.22 Power Squat*

Fig.23 High Half-Kneel Stance

The manoeuvre:

▶ Communicate clearly and appropriately with the individual and/or colleague(s);
▶ Identify who will lead any team move;
▶ Agree on the words of command (e.g., 'Ready, steady, slide');
▶ Carry out the move while ensuring that it is controlled and smooth;
▶ Use transfer of body weight to achieve a move and not a stationery stance with pulling or pushing using the arms;
▶ Ensure the individual is left in a safe and comfortable position;
▶ Review the manoeuvre, checking that the move went as expected and if it did not, report and record your concerns.

Appropriate holds

Inappropriate holds and grips can be harmful, causing pain, discomfort or bruising. The following techniques can be used to eliminate or reduce the risk of harm from inappropriate holds and grips:

▶ Where possible use an open palm, keeping fingers and thumb together, and place the palm on to the individual (see fig. 24 and fig. 25)

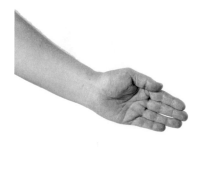 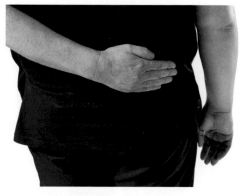

Fig.24   *Fig.25*

▶ Where an individual's hand needs to be held then use a palm to palm hold without locking thumbs (see fig. 26 on the next page)

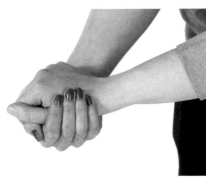

Fig.26

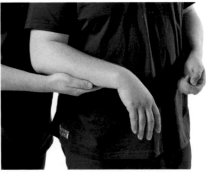

Fig.27

➡ If someone has a weak arm it can be supported under the forearm, do not support directly under the elbow as you may apply undue pressure to the shoulder joint (see fig. 27)

➡ Long arm support gives more control (see fig. 28)

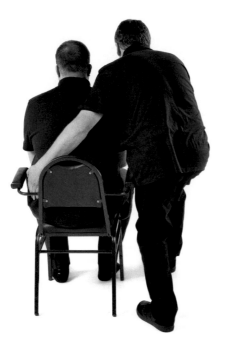

Fig.28

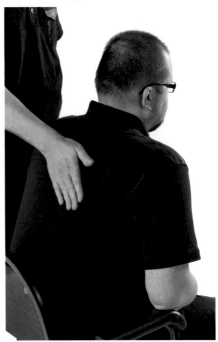

Fig.29

⏩ The central key point gives lighter, touch-prompt assistance (see fig. 29)

⏩ Support in front of the shoulder can help an individual stabilise and balance when standing (see fig. 30)

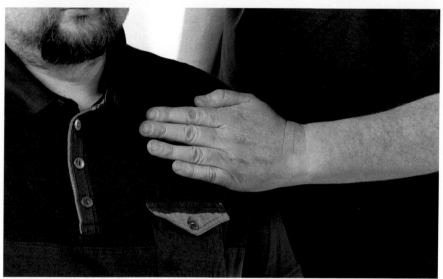

Fig 30

Unit 12
Basic Stance

If the stance described below and its associated principles are applied during all manual handling activities, the stresses to your back will be significantly reduced with obvious resulting benefits.

The Stance

Face Forward – this will align the back by having feet, hips, shoulders and head pointing the same way.

Walk Stance – this will create a stable base over which you can transfer your weight.

Flex – moderate flexion through your whole body.

Transfer Body Weight – allow your weight to travel over your base in order to move a load.

Where you need the stance at a lower level then a high, half-kneel stance can be used as this still allows for the application of the principles of Face Forward, Walk Stance, Flexion and Transfer Body Weight. Protect your knees by using a kneel pad when on hard surfaces.

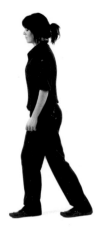
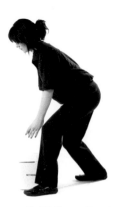
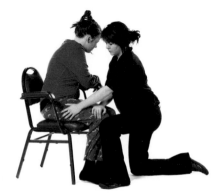

Fig.31 Walk Stance   *Fig.32 Power Squat*   *Fig.33 High Half-Kneel Stance*

Face Forward does not necessarily mean that you will move in a forward direction, sometimes you will be moving backwards while your body is in the Face Forward position.

Basic stance for pulling and pushing:

➡ Adopt the basic stance above;
➡ Let your body weight and leg muscles do the work;
➡ Keep your elbows close to your side and slightly bent;
➡ Once the load is moving, continue by pushing through your feet;
➡ A walking upright position should be adopted as soon as possible.

For pulling: start with your weight on your front foot and transfer your weight on to your back foot as you control the load. Leaning your weight in this way allows your body weight to do most of the work rather than pulling with your arms as this could strain the neck and shoulders (see fig. 34)

For pushing: start with your weight on your back foot and transfer your weight on to your front foot as you control the load (i.e., the reverse of the pulling action) (see fig. 35)

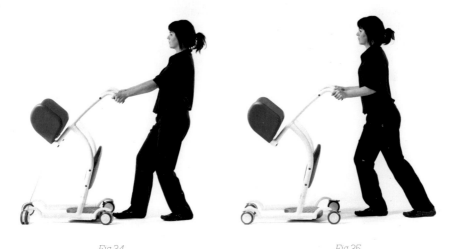

Fig 34   Fig 35

This technique can be adopted for any pull or push action such as pushing a hoist or pulling on a slide sheet.

Pushing or pulling as a team

Using the techniques described above:

➡ Adjust the height of the work surface to a comfortable working height before starting. (If a team member has a significant height difference from the rest of the team then it may be better for them not to participate);

➡ One person should plan, coordinate and give the commands for the move;

➡ Several small moves are often more desirable than trying to complete the whole movement in one go;

➡ Involve as many people as the move requires (i.e. ASSESS).

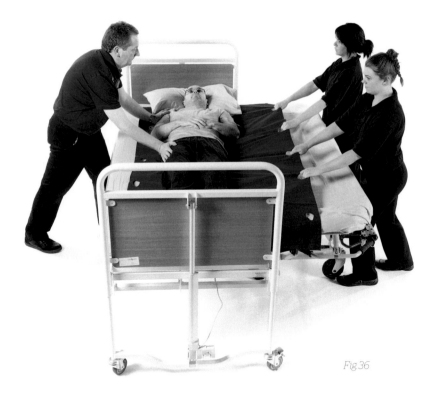

Fig 36

Research has demonstrated that moderate flexion throughout the whole body, including the back, is more beneficial than focusing solely on flexing the knees (as when you bend your knees and keep your back straight (the alignment of the back is better described as 'spine in line maintaining its natural curves')).

A power squat is preferable to a straight up and down movement as it uses moderate flexion and allows the person moving to move forward on to his or her front foot as he or she stands, which allows a natural movement pattern.

For the manual handling of people this stance can be adopted to facilitate all the movement techniques required. Once the stance and associated movement patterns are learned, it can become the automatic position adopted by the lifter, allowing the lifter to focus attention on the individual requiring assistance rather than on himself or herself. Whilst other stances are not necessarily incorrect, the fewer that have to be learnt the quicker the basic stance can be assimilated and so if this basic stance enables lifters to adopt a good position while assisting individuals to move, why learn any others?

Along with the stance other principles need to be considered and applied where relevant; these are:

➡ Assessing the situation using TILE;
➡ Keeping the load as close to the body as possible;
➡ Considering the centre of gravity of the load in relation to your own;
➡ Establishing a suitable hold for appropriate control and support;
➡ Using feet to change direction;
➡ Giving clear instruction if others involved;
➡ Ensuring the movement is controlled and smooth, and not sudden and jerky.

Unit 13
General Use of Equipment

Equipment Used In Manual Handling

Equipment can be used to reduce the risks involved in manual handling operations provided that:

a) A risk assessment has been undertaken.
b) Staff have been appropriately trained in equipment's use.
c) Equipment is safe to use, properly maintained and clean.

When using equipment, account must also be taken of the individual's tissue viability and infection control.

> All equipment must be visually inspected by staff prior to use. If anything is found to be defective, the equipment must immediately be withdrawn from service and the defect brought to the attention of an appropriate person.

Keypoints For Manual Handling Equipment

All equipment should:

- Be appropriate for the task, user, individual and environment;
- Be assessed as suitable for the task, user, individual and environment (and this should be recorded on the individual's Handling Assessment);
- Be properly maintained and serviced;
- Be visually checked and confirmed as safe and in a good state of repair prior to every use;
- Be removed from use if found faulty in any way and reported as such;
- Only be used by staff who have received training in its use and the risks associated with its use;

➡ Be used in accordance with the manufacturer's instructions;
➡ Only be used following a manual handling assessment of the individual's needs which has also taken account of:

  ➡ Safe working load;
  ➡ Tissue viability;
  ➡ Pressure area care;
  ➡ Infection control.

> All equipment is useful in the correctly assessed circumstances
> AND
> ALL equipment is hazardous if used inappropriately or
> when incorrectly assessed.

Pushing equipment

When pushing equipment always take the following steps:

1. Check equipment is suitable for the move and is safe and clean to use.
2. Check brakes work and wheels are running smoothly.
3. Take a comfortable hold – preferably with two hands in front of you with elbows slightly bent (a hoist can be held at any point on the handle, allowing you to push or pull with your body weight without twisting) (see fig. 37 and fig. 38)

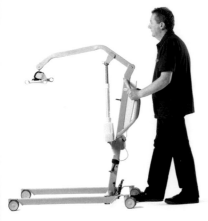
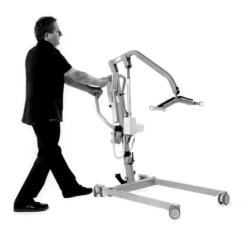

Fig. 37

Fig. 38

4. Adopt the basic push stance with your weight on the back foot.
5. Lean your weight into the direction of the move (see fig. 39) and avoid twisting as you move; several small moves backwards and forwards to reposition the wheels will assist the movement.

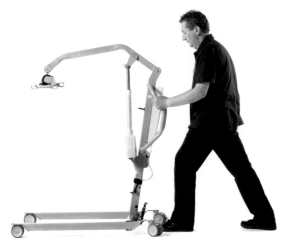

Fig.39

6. Once the move is initiated, keep the movement going by coming up into a walk stance and pushing through your feet as you walk (see fig. 37 on the previus page)
7. In order to turn set the wheels in the direction of the movement (see fig. 40 and fig. 41)

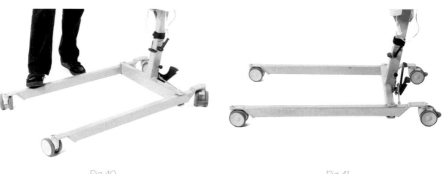

Fig 40   Fig 41

Pulling equipment

As for pushing but:

1. Adopt the basic pull stance with your weight on the front foot.
2. Lean your weight into the direction of the move (see fig. 42)
3. Once the move is initiated keep the movement going by coming up into a walk stance and pushing through your feet as you walk (be aware of what is around you if you are going backwards).

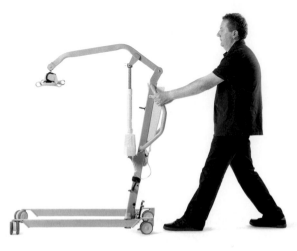

Fig 42

Management Of A Profile Bed

When the head section of a profile bed is raised, the individual may be 'pushed' down the bed. This will result in the individual being left in a position that is uncomfortable and in which it will be difficult for them to breathe or drink; their tissue viability will also be compromised by friction and shearing as they are pushed down the bed.

The main cause of an individual being pushed down the bed is the contact of his or her back with the bed.

To prevent this, the following steps should be taken:

➡ Place a small slide sheet behind the individual's back or have an in-bed slide system in situ.
➡ Raise the head section of the profile bed until the individual is at an angle of about 45°.Raise the knee section to a comfortable position (see fig. 43)
➡ Complete raising the head section until the individual is comfortable.
➡ Once the individual's back has slid up the back rest as the profile is raised, remove the slide sheet.
➡ Ensure the individual is comfortable.

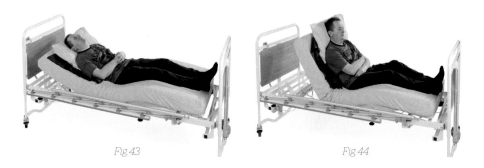

Fig 43   Fig 44

(Occasionally some assistance may be necessary: if so, simply adjust the slide sheet in the direction of the top of the bed (see fig. 44)

Alternatively, if no slide sheet is available:

➡ As the back rest is raised, ask the individual to rock his or her shoulders one at a time thus lifting them clear of the bed and allowing their body to move up the bed (see fig. 45)

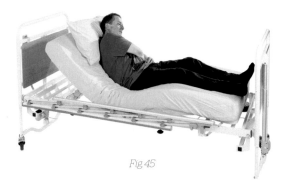

Fig 45

Slide gloves

Slide gloves (see fig. 46) can be used as an aid when a slide sheet is being used for small movements and adjustments such as:

- Moving feet across the bed (in this case, place your hand with the slide glove on under the individual's feet. Do not lift the feet, but have your hand resting on the bed and the individual's feet resting on your gloved hand and then slide the feet into position;
- Inserting a sling, to ease and smooth the sling into place (see fig. 47)

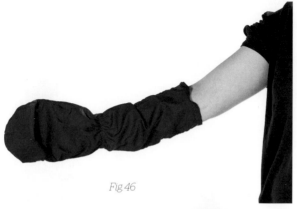

Fig 46

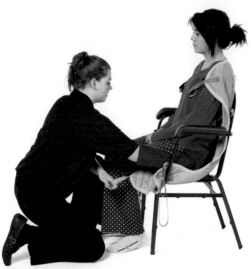

Fig 47

Transfer or handling belts

Transfer belts should:

➡ Be used with caution by properly trained personnel;

➡ Be assessed as suitable for the individual and the activity;

➡ Fit closely around the waist area but not be too tight;

➡ Be held by taking hold of a loop (but do not put your hand through the loop) (see fig. 48)

➡ NOT be used to lift an individual, for example, up from a chair or the floor;

➡ NOT be used to hold an individual up when standing if they are falling.

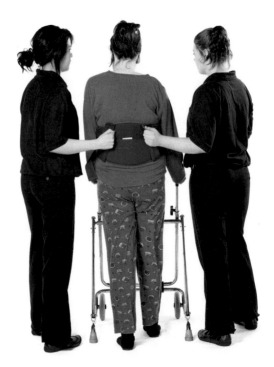

Fig 48

Unit 14
Use of Hoists and Slings

Hoists

A hoist is a device that mechanically lifts an individual. There are many types of hoist, but they can be divided for convenience into two main categories:

Active hoists – standing, these hoists are designed to help an individual stand or move; as such, their use presupposes some functional capacity in the individual, including in particular the capacity to bear weight and the ability to balance while standing (see fig. 49)

Passive hoists – these, when used with an appropriate sling, may be employed to lift an individual who has no ability to stand. They will be either mobile or overhead track hoists (see fig. 50)

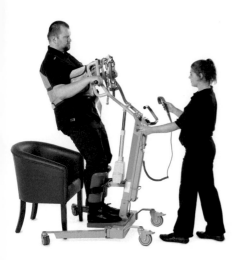

Fig 49

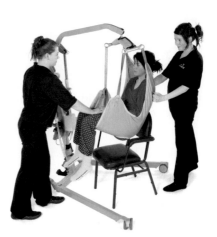

Fig 50

The spreader bar

Passive hoists come in a range of spreader types which either allow for a loop-sling attachment or a clip attachment (see fig. 51). The spreader may be in a 'coathanger' style, a four point or a 'wishbone' style. It is important that the sling chosen is compatible with the hoist and spreader.

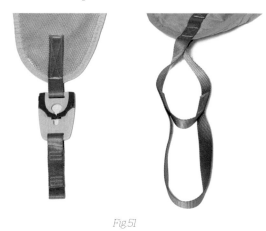

Fig 51

SLINGS

It is critical that the individual to be moved is assessed by a competent person who can decide on both the style and size of sling required. If there are options for positioning or a choice of loops, then this also should be assessed. Once the correct choice has been made, it should be recorded on the individual's manual handling plan as part of the system of work for carers to follow.

Standing aid hoist slings

Standard standing aid hoist slings provide support behind the individual's back and are used to bring the individual up into a standing position (see fig. 52)
Transport slings give some support to the individual's legs, allowing the individual to half sit in the sling, and give more support to the individual who has erratic standing ability. Nevertheless, the individual will still be using some functional capacity in his or her legs and upper body.

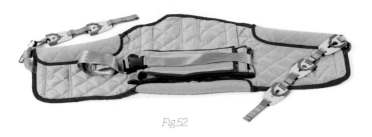

Fig 52

Passive hoist slings

There are three common shapes or styles of sling which will suit many individuals who need hoisting.

Toilet/Access sling: these give good access for the removal of clothing for toilet and hygiene purposes. However, they do not give sufficient support for some individuals and careful assessment is required. These slings are unlikely to be suitable for individuals with poor cognition, low tone, spasm or a tendency to seizures and some individuals find they cause discomfort behind the thighs (see fig. 53 and fig. 54)

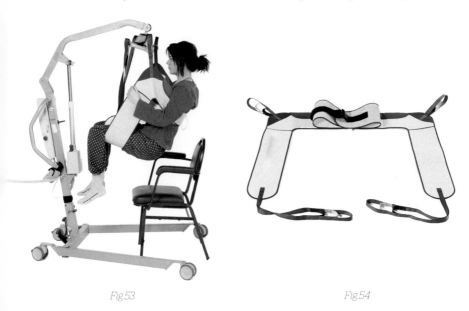

Fig 53   *Fig 54*

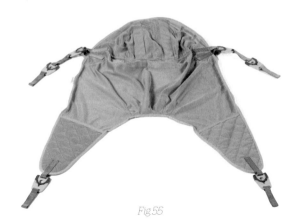

Fig 55

Quickfit/Universal style: these are easy to fit and give more support than an access sling but less than a deluxe version (see fig. 55). Some individuals will need head support during hoisting and if this is the case, a sling with head support should be used; alternatively a neck roll may be suitable.

Deluxe/divided leg hammock style: these give greater support and comfort during the lift and can also have a head support if required (see fig. 56).

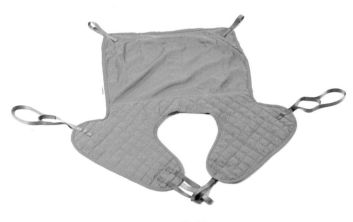

Fig 56

Specialist styles: some individuals require specialised support in order to be lifted safely and comfortably. Examples of this would be:

- Amputee slings;
- Hammock slings (with or without a commode aperture).
- Standing harness (these are often seen in therapy settings and can be used to support an individual to stand who has difficulty bearing weight).

Standard Elements for the Use of Hoists and Slings

Ensure the hoist and sling have been assessed as suitable for:

- The task to be undertaken (e.g., bathing, lifts from the floor etc);
- The individual (size, style, material, support given, etc);
- The load (i.e., a safe working load);
- The working environment (overhead tracking gantry / mobile);
- Use with other equipment   (i.e., given the other equipment present, is the individual accessible for the hoist and sling and is the hoist and sling compatible with this equipment);
- The user (ease of use, ease of pushing (flooring, caster type, handles)).

Key points for choosing a hoist:

- Does it meet the needs of the individual?
- Is it appropriate for the tasks required?
- Is it appropriate for the user?
- Is it appropriate for the environment?
- Does it need to support the full or partial bodyweight of the individual?
- Is the individual's weight within the safe capacity/working load of the hoist?
- Is it in good working order and correctly maintained?

REPORT any equipment that is found to be faulty
or that malfunctions while being used.

REMOVE such equipment from use or put a notice on it
that indicates that it is faulty.

Hoist and Sling: Inspection Before Use

The checklist below is intended as a guide and there may be additional features of the users particular hoist and sling which should also be inspected – check with the product manufacturer.

As well as being inspected by the user, the hoist and sling must be properly maintained and formally inspected every six months or with compliance with the manufacturer's manual.

Hoist

Check that:

- There is no missing hardware or broken pieces;
- The battery is charged;
- The base opens and closes easily;
- There is no looseness in casters and bolts;
- The casters swivel and roll smoothly;
- The casters are clean (e.g., no dust or hair impedes their action);
- There are no cracks in or deflections of the mast and/or boom and they are not loose;
- The boom is centered properly between the base legs;
- There is no wear in or damage to the spreader or swivel bar bolts and sling hooks;
- There is no wear in or damage to the spreader or swivel bar joint with the boom;
- The hoist is bearing a safe working load.

Sling

Check that:

- There are no signs of wear or deterioration in the sling material;
- There is no wear in the sling straps, d-rings or plastic clips for attachment to the hoist spreader;
- There are no defects or loose threads in the stitched areas;
- The sling has been cleaned in accordance with the manufacturer's instructions;
- Any labelling is clear and legible;
- The sling is bearing a safe working load and in particular that the size of the load does not exceed safety limits;
- The sling is compatible with the hoist.

Key points for using hoists

Ensure the individual's specific handling plan is read and followed.
And check the hoist for wear and tear and cleanliness.
If in doubt: do not use and report your doubts.

➡ Follow the manufacturer's instructions and the individuals handling plan;
➡ Plan the situation;
➡ Use the correct type and size of sling (i.e. the type specified in the individual's handling plan and recommended by the manufacturer);
➡ Do not combine one manufacturer's sling with another manufacturer's hoist without prior arrangement or a compatibility statement;
➡ Have as many carers present as the situation requires (e.g., commonly two carers when using a mobile hoist but often only one carer when using an overhead hoist). Assess each individual and situation and then record your decision on the individual's handling plan;
➡ Make sure that the individual is adequately supervised and supported during the transfer. Consider having a carer stay by the individual's side, or hold the sling, during the transfer while a second carer moves the hoist (see fig. 57)
➡ Remember that the hoist need not be brought directly towards the individual but can be brought from a slightly oblique angle (see fig. 58), which will be less intimidating to the individual and leaves space in front of him or her for the carer to apply the sling and maintain good communication with the individual;

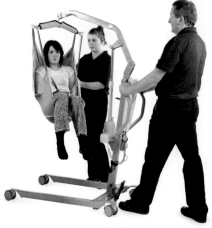
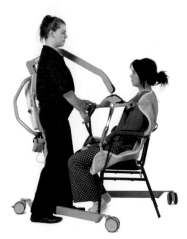

Fig.57   *Fig.58*

➡ Remember that an oblique approach when hoisting from the floor will bring the spreader to an optimum position. Ensure that the individual has his or her head on a pillow and a carer beside him or her (see fig. 59)

➡ When approaching a seated individual, either keep the spreader bar as low as possible (ideally below the individual's shoulder level) or above his or her head and then lowering before attaching the sling (see fig. 58 on the previous page)

➡ Transfer the individual the shortest distance possible and where a significant distance is unavoidable, transfer the individual to a wheelchair and rehoist him or her at the arrival point;

➡ When hoisting from a profile bed lift the individual from a sitting position where possible (see fig. 60) but if the individual must be lifted from a lying position ensure he or she receives suitable head support from the sling;

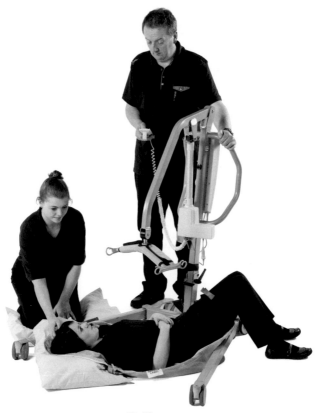

Fig 59

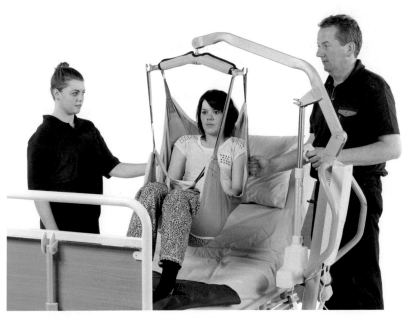

Fig 60

⮕ Use your body weight to slowly push and pull the hoist; lean your weight slowly in the direction of your movement. Remember fast pulling or pushing will significantly raise the effort required from you;

⮕ To turn the hoist round, always hold the handle but remember you can pull it towards you or push it away from the side rather than going behind the mast and twisting it round (see chapter on General Use of Equipment fig. 39 and fig. 42)

⮕ Always set the wheels in the direction of movement before changing the direction of the hoist (i.e., parallel wheels are set for movement straight forward or back; wheels are set as if in a circle for turning (see chapter on General Use of Equipment fig. 40 and fig. 41)

⮕ Remember, in general, the brakes are NOT applied for raising or lowering an individual from a chair or bed; the final decision whether or not to apply the brakes will come from a specific assessment of the situation;

⮕ NEVER pull the sling and individual out of the hoist's base or centre of gravity during a lift or lowering as this could destablilise the hoist.

Transfer from chair, bed or the floor using a hoist

➔ Collect the correct sling and check it is clean and safe to use;

➔ Check the hoist is in good working order and the battery is charged;

➔ Communicate throughout the transfer;

➔ Maintain dignity and privacy during the move.

The handler and assist as follows

➔ Apply the sling (a sling with head support should be used when lifting from a lying position);

➔ Widen the base of the hoist and position the hoist correctly in relation to the individual (see fig. 61, fig. 62 and fig. 63)

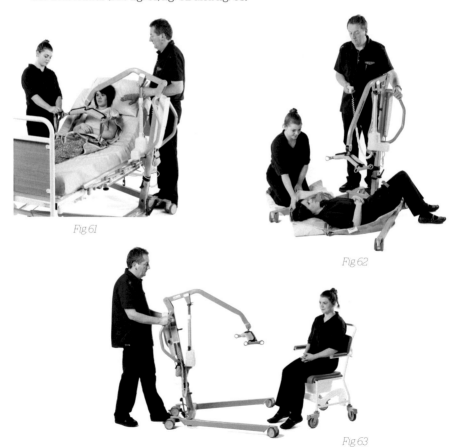

Fig. 61

Fig 62

Fig 63

- ➡ Attach the sling to the spreader bar (see fig. 64)
- ➡ Check the brakes are off;
- ➡ Raise the individual until they are clear of the surface;
- ➡ Close the base of the hoist;
- ➡ Ensure individual is comfortable and secure (this may require a carer to be by his or her side during the transfer and even holding the sling) (see fig. 16 on the page 35 and fig. 60 on the page 67)
- ➡ Move the hoist smoothly and slowly to the destination, opening the base as required;
- ➡ Ensure the individual is correctly positioned over the destination and lower;
- ➡ Detach the sling from the spreader bar;
- ➡ Move hoist away from the individual;
- ➡ Remove the sling by turning the leg pieces under themselves and peeling out (see fig. 65 and fig. 66)

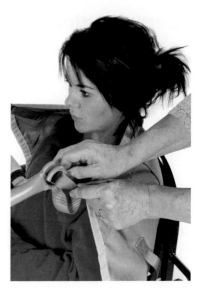

Fig 64

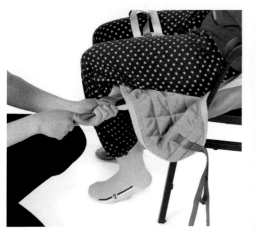

Fig 65

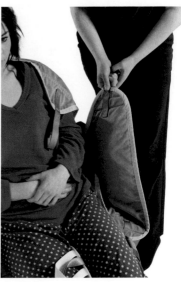

Fig 66

Inserting a sling in a chair

Ensure that the individual's specific individual handling plan has been read and is followed. Check the sling for wear and tear and cleanliness: if in doubt do not use and report.

➡ Ask the individual to lean forward slightly, if they cannot do this, a second carer could support the individual's forward movement of the shoulders;

➡ Slide the sling down behind the individual's back (see fig. 67) until the base edge meets the seat of the chair. (It is important to get the centre of the sling right down or else the sling will not pass around the bottom and support the individual effectively. This can be made easier by holding the leg part of the sling firmly with one hand creating some resistance for the other hand to push against (see fig. 68) as it slides down the back: a slide glove will make this easier);

➡ Ease the side of the sling down by each hip;

➡ Where possible, ask the individual to lean to one side;

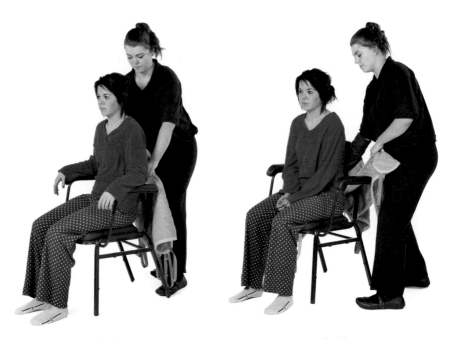

Fig 67   Fig 68

➡ Adopt a comfortable position in front of the individual and, taking care not to stoop, hold the leg piece firmly in one hand and pull it forward as the other hand eases the sling under the individual's hip and buttock. (see fig. 69)

➡ Repeat for the other hip;

➡ Raise the individual's leg by placing the foot on your thigh (placing a towel or paper sheet on your leg) and pass the sling under the thigh (see fig. 70)

➡ Repeat on the other side;

➡ Ensure the leg pieces are placed according to the sling instructions; however, commonly one leg strap is passed through the other so that the leg pieces cannot separate during the lift. Alternatively there may be a strap on one of the leg pieces which allows the other leg piece to be passed through. (see fig. 71) The leg pieces should be just behind the knee once fitted.

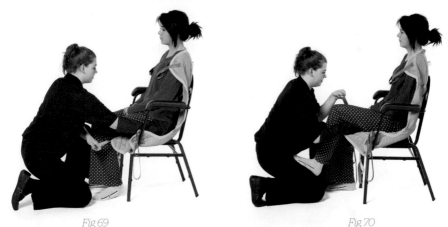

Fig 69   Fig 70

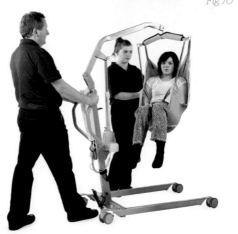

Fig 71

Inserting a sling on the bed or floor

Ensure the individual's specific handling plan has been read and is followed. Check the sling for wear and tear and cleanliness: if in doubt do not use and report.

The application of a sling should not require the individual to be turned on to his or her side more than once: additional turns can be stressful and invasive as well as requiring the carer to undertake more manual handling.

If the individual can tolerate side lying unsupported then a single carer can apply the sling; if not a second carer should be positioned on the opposite side of the individual. If a single carer is applying the sling on a bed then it may be necessary to raise a safety/bed rail on the opposite side of the bed to ensure safety during the task.

⊡ Hold the sling with the outside/labels facing the handler (do not lay the sling on the floor or bed at this stage) (see fig. 72)
⊡ Lay the sling over the individual at the correctly measured position (e.g., lower edge at coccyx);
⊡ Allow the remaining sling material to lie flat across the floor or bed surface;
⊡ Take hold of the edge of the sling that is lying on the floor or bed surface and roll it up so that the roll is on top of the sling (see fig. 73)

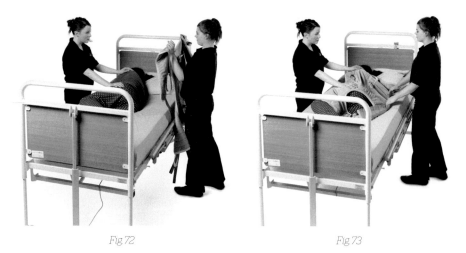

Fig. 72   Fig. 73

⊡ Find the midpoint of the sling at the neck edge and find the individual's cervical vertebrae and place the two points together;

➡ Hold the sling in this position and smooth the excess material over the individual's shoulder, then tuck the roll under the individual's shoulder so that it cannot unroll (see fig. 74)

➡ Pass the shoulder strap under the pillow to facilitate removal later;

➡ Find the midpoint of the sling at the bottom edge and place in line with the individual's buttock crease;

➡ Hold the sling in position with one hand; smooth any excess material over the individual and tuck the roll under the individual's hip to prevent it unrolling. (see fig. 75) Place the leg straps as close to the leg as possible;

➡ Ask the individual to roll on to his or her back, assisting if necessary;

➡ Take hold of the shoulder strap from under the pillow and draw the sling through. With the other hand palm upwards, find the edge of the roll and unroll as the sling is drawn through (see fig. 76)

➡ Continue to draw the sling through until all is lying flat on the bed;

➡ Place the leg pieces under the individual's legs ready for attachment to the hoist.

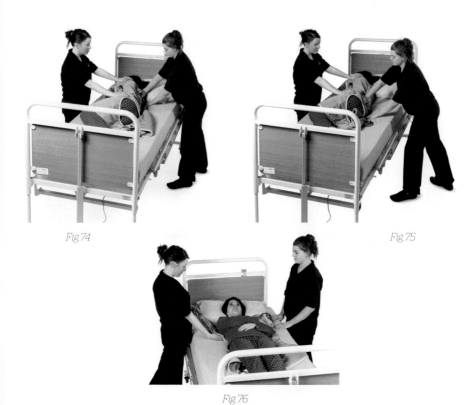

Fig. 74

Fig. 75

Fig. 76

Inserting a sling with slide sheets for an individual who cannot roll

▶ Insert a pair of flat slide sheets under the individual (see chapter Use of Slide Sheets);

▶ Lay the sling alongside the individual's side;

▶ Pass the shoulder strap under the pillow between the two slide sheets;

▶ Pass the leg strap under the knee and ease the sling across the bed as far as is easily possible;

▶ Ease the shoulder section of the sling between the two slide sheets until it is just under the nearer shoulder (see fig. 77)

▶ Either raise a safe bed rail and go round to the other side of the bed or, if a second carer is present, he or she can proceed to draw the sling through gently;

▶ Using the shoulder and leg straps, gradually ease the sling under the individual until it is in the right position;

▶ Check the sling is in the correct position (if a leg piece is held out to the side of the bed, the edge will be in line with the base of the sling) (see fig. 78)

▶ If the sling needs to be brought further down the body, do this by holding the leg piece and pulling in a diagonal direction down the bed (see fig. 79)

▶ Repeat from the other side;

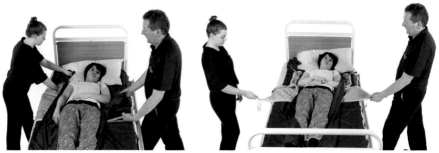

Fig 77   Fig 78

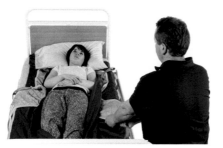

Fig 79

➡ Once the sling is correctly fitted then remove the slide sheets (see fig. 80)

➡ Elevate the back of the bed so that the individual is hoisted from a sitting position (see fig. 81) If the individual has to be hoisted from a lying position he or she should have a sling with head support or a neck roll fitted.

If the individual is sitting up in bed, the sling can be applied in the same way as for sitting in a chair.

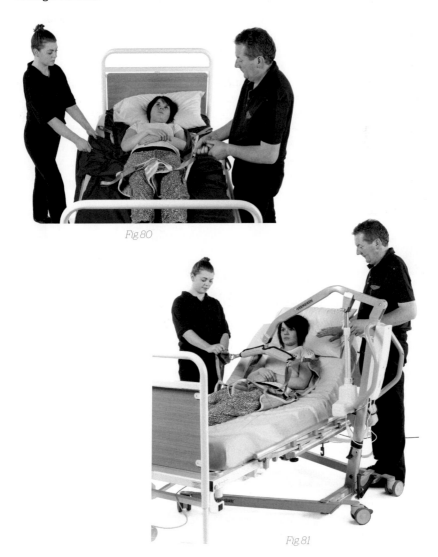

Fig 80

Fig 81

Positions for hoisting individuals

Every individual should be assessed for his or her optimum transfer position. The risks to the individual during a transfer can be reduced by ensuring he or she is not in too upright a position during movement and that additionally a carer is close by at all times to reduce anxiety and excessive movement. The carer can hold the sling to stabilise the individual during the transfer.

A semi-reclined position (see fig. 82) is often the position of choice for transfers as it takes the pressure off the back of the legs and may be more comfortable; additionally it is harder for the individual to tip forward or sideways out of the sling.

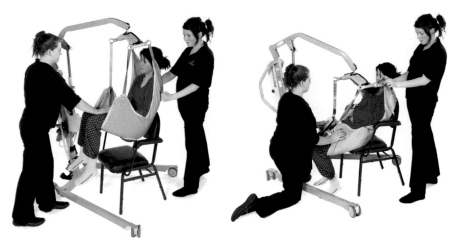

Fig 82   Fig 83

A reclined position spreads the weight across the back of the individual and again reduces pressure on the back of the legs. The individual will need head support on the sling or a neck roll. This position is often used for an amputee or hammock style slings.

Upright positions are the most vulnerable as the individual may tip forward or sideways out of the sling, particularly if there is any swinging during the transfer. Swinging can be reduced by a carer holding the sling and individual during the move. An upright position may be desirable for positioning the individual well in his or her chair but this can be achieved after the transfer and once the individual is over the seat, using the following approach:

➡ Lower the individual on to the seating;
➡ Ensure the individual cannot slip forward (see fig. 83)

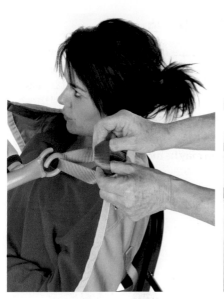 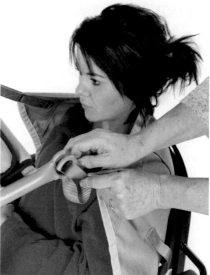

Fig 84   *Fig 85*

➡ Attach a short loop from the shoulder strap on to the spreader (it is not necessary to remove the initial loop) (see fig. 84 and fig. 85)

➡ Raise the individual until they are just clear of the seating, guide to the back of the chair and immediately lower again on to the chair (see fig. 86) (the carer can assist by pushing on the sling as the individual is lowered).

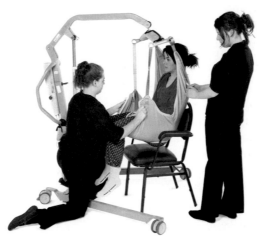

Fig 86

To remove a sling

From a seated position:

➡ Turn the leg strap under itself and peel away from the individual's leg;
➡ Repeat for the other leg strap (see fig. 87)
➡ Lean the individual forward and slide the sling up and out.

From a lying position:

➡ Roll one edge of the sling close to the individual's body with the roll next to the bed;
➡ Turn the individual to lie on his or her side and draw the sling through and out.

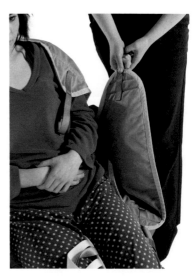

Fig 87

Using a standing aid hoist

Ensure the individual's specific handling plan has been read and is followed. Check the hoist and sling for wear and tear and cleanliness: if in doubt do not use and report. The individual should have some weight-bearing ability and standing balance as this hoist is an 'active' and not a 'passive' lifter.

➡ One or two carers may be needed, depending on the individual's needs, and this should be recorded on the individual's handling plan;
➡ If two carers are present one must stay by the individual at all times and ensure his or her comfort and safety;
➡ Apply the hoist sling behind the individual's back;
➡ Open the base of the hoist;
➡ Bring the hoist in towards the individual and ask him or her to place his or her feet on the footplate (see fig. 88)
➡ Brakes can be applied, if required, at this stage and during the stand but should remain off when lowering the individual back into a sitting position;
➡ Attach the assessed loop on to the spreader bar;
➡ Ask the individual to hold on to the handle position of the hoist and to push through the feet during the stand;
➡ Raise the individual to a standing position (see fig. 89) do not stop with the individual in a squat position as this is very hard for them to maintain and can cause discomfort;

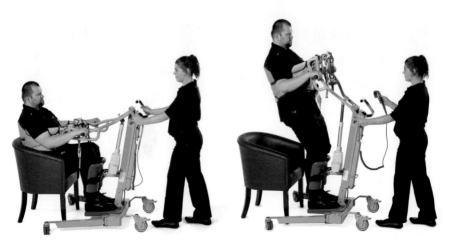

Fig 88   Fig 89

➡ Check the hoist sling has not slid up into the individual's axilla. (There should be room to place a couple of fingers between the top edge of the sling and the individual's axilla (see fig. 90). If the sling is right up in the axilla then report and ask for a reassessment as it could be an indication that the individual is not weight-bearing sufficiently and they may require a passive lifting hoist);

➡ Move the hoist away from the furniture and close the base of the hoist;

➡ Transfer the individual to the destination position (this should be a short distance transfer only unless a transport sling is being used);

➡ Open the base, position the individual over the destination, check brakes are off and lower the individual;

➡ Detach the sling and remove both the hoist and sling;

➡ Ensure the individual is safe and comfortable.

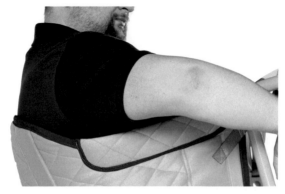

Fig 90

Unit 15
Use of Slide Sheets

Standard Elements

➡ Check that the slide sheet has been assessed as suitable for the individual's needs, that it is clean and safe to use and that you have been trained in its use;

➡ Check that the slide sheet covers the whole bed (see fig. 91) or is long enough to be placed under all the contact points of the person and allows for the distance of the move (see fig. 92), also consider using two smaller slide sheets (see fig. 93)

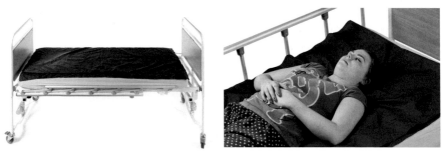

Fig 91   Fig 92

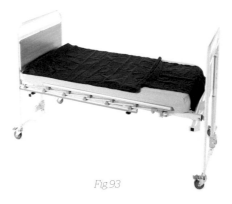

Fig 93

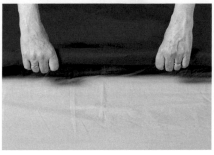 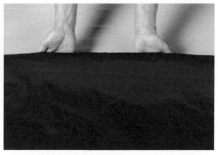

Fig 94   Fig 95

➡ If the individual's head is on a pillow, place the slide sheet under the pillow;

➡ Adjust the bed to a height suitable for the activity and the height of the carers;

➡ Insert slide sheet under all contact points of the individual;

➡ To insert slide sheets roll up and place the roll next to the bed (see fig. 94) so that it can easily be brought through by placing your hand, palm up, under the roll and pulling through (see fig. 95). (This method allows the individual to only have to roll once into side lying);

➡ When using, hold the top sheet, or top surface of the sheet, only, either using handles or holding the sheet. (see fig. 96 and fig. 97)

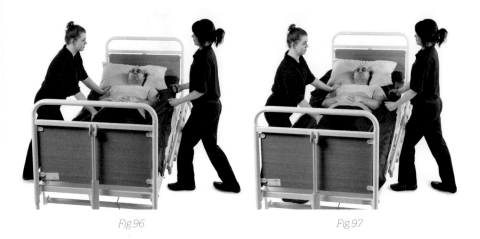

Fig 96   Fig 97

➡ Hold at a significant contact point (i.e. shoulder/hip or both).

➡ Keep wrist in a neutral position if possible with hands in front or close to the body:

▶ To complete a move, stand in the basic stance along the line of the intended move (i.e., obliquely by looking at the bottom opposite corner of the bed or facing down or across the bed, depending on which direction you wish to move). Make sure you are:

  ▶ Flexed;
  ▶ Face forward (i.e. spine in line);
  ▶ In walk stance ('tug of war' position);
  ▶ With weight on the front foot.

▶ Complete the move by transferring weight from your front foot on to your back foot as you bring the individual towards you;

▶ Make sure your move is smooth, controlled and slow;

▶ Consider whether two short movements are preferable to trying to complete the move in one movement;

▶ Remove the slide sheet by turning one corner underneath the slide sheet and drawing slowly out, keeping the slide sheet as flat as possible rather than bunching it as this can cause discomfort (see fig. 98)

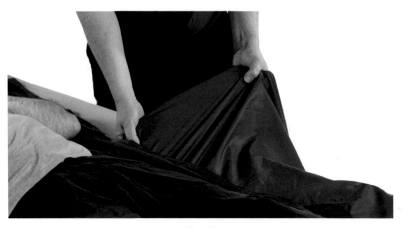

Fig 98

For all the moves ensure the following have been considered:

The environment/equipment

▶ Adjust the bed to an appropriate working height;

▶ Ensure the brakes on the bed are on;

▶ Check the slide sheet is the right size and safe and clean to use.

The individual

➡ Explain the process to the individual and seek his or her consent to proceed;
➡ Ensure you are working in accordance with the individual's manual handling plan;
➡ Ensure the individual lies flat with one pillow between him or her and the slide sheet, or no pillow as required;
➡ Ensure all the individual's contact points are on the slide sheet

Inserting slide sheets

These methods can be used for both roller slide sheets and pairs of flat slide sheets.

For an individual who can roll

a) With the individual already in side lying position:

➡ Roll up approximately a third of the top half of the slide sheet/s (see fig. 99)
➡ Lay this roll against the individual's back and ease the edge just under the back. Make sure the individual's head is on the slide sheet; if a pillow is in place then the slide sheet should be underneath it (see fig. 100)
➡ Roll up approximately a third of the remaining slide sheet and smooth just under the hip and well under the legs and feet (see fig. 101 on the next page)
➡ Ask or assist the individual to turn on to his or her back;
➡ With palms up and using your fingers gradually unroll the slide sheet from under the individual (see fig. 102 on the next page)

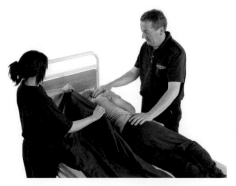

Fig 99

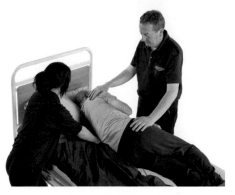

Fig 100

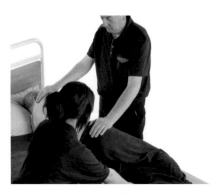

Fig.101

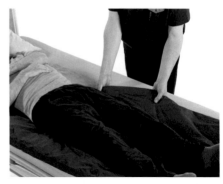

Fig.102

b) With person lying flat:

➡ Roll up approximately two thirds of the slide sheet/s (it is easier to work with the head-end first and then the lower end, rather than trying to do it all in one go);

➡ Lay this roll against the individual's side and ease the edge just under the head, back and legs (see fig. 103). Make sure the individual's head is on the slide sheet; if a pillow is in place then the slide sheet should be underneath it;

➡ Ask the individual to lie on his or her side, or assist him or her to do so;

➡ With palms up and using your fingers, gradually unroll the slide sheet from under the individual (see fig. 104)

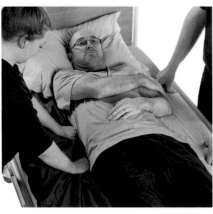

Fig.103

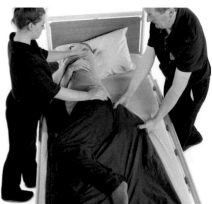

Fig.104

For an individual who cannot roll and with two carers:

▶ Each carer take hold of one side of the slide sheet;

▶ Together roll a panel of slide sheet and continue until almost all of the slide sheet is rolled (see fig. 105)

▶ Place the rolled slide sheet under the individual's pillow, ensuring the rolled panel is next to the bed;

▶ Standing on either side of the bed, adopt the basic stance facing the head of the bed;

▶ With the nearside hands and palms up, grasp the panel (see fig. 106) and together pull the slide sheet down the bed by unrolling the panel in sections (see fig. 107). Keep tension across the bed to ensure the slide sheet stays flat.

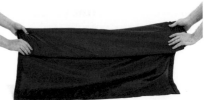

Fig 105

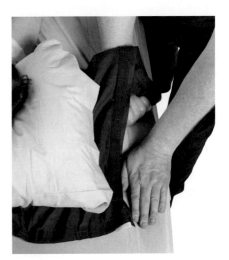

Fig 106

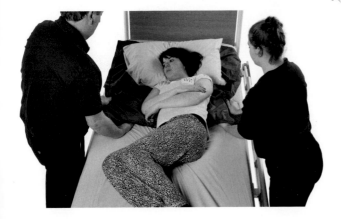

Fig 107

Removing slide sheets

- ➡ Find one corner of the slide sheet/s;
- ➡ Pass this corner under the slide sheet and draw the slide sheet across, up and out from under the individual (see fig. 108)
- ➡ For comfort keep the slide sheet flat; do not 'bunch it up' as it is drawn out;
- ➡ Remove flat sheets either singly or together;
- ➡ Use this method for all slide sheets.

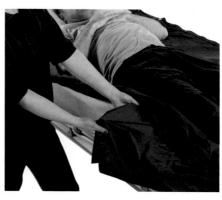

Fig.108

Repositioning A Person In Bed

Moving Up The Bed

- ➡ Ideally for this move the bed should be flat. The individual should lie flat with a pillow between him or her and the slide sheet, although this is not essential (a pillow controls the head and neck during the move and can be more comfortable; it also reduces the noise of the slide sheet against the individual's head). It is acceptable for the individual to be in a semi-reclined position but the bed angle must not exceed approximately 20° of tilt (see fig. 109). Lowering the head end of

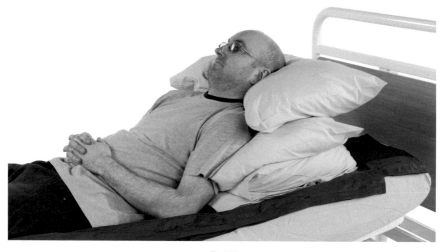

Fig.109

the bed (i.e., a reverse Trendelenberg position) can be used to gravity assist the slide but the individual's medical condition must have been assessed beforehand as suitable for this move and the bed tilt should not exceed 30°. This move generally requires two handlers although one handler can execute the move as long as the individual's capability has been assessed and the individual's weight is not significantly more than that of the carer doing the moving.

Assist as follows:

▶ Insert the slide sheet under the individual, ensuring all points of contact are on the slide sheet (i.e. under head, trunk and feet (an in-bed sliding and repositioning system can be used, thus eliminating the need for slide sheets to be inserted));
▶ Stand on either side of the bed, at the head end (the handler/s can stand behind the pillow at the top of the bed if there is no headboard);
▶ Face the opposite bottom corner of the bed (see fig. 110) (oblique position) or straight down the bed (see fig. 111)

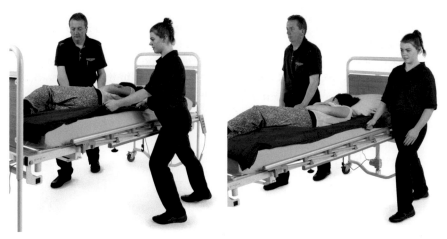

Fig 110   Fig 111

▶ Adopt the basic, base walk-stance of feet slightly apart and one foot in advance of the other;
▶ Hold the top layer of slide sheet by the individual's shoulder or shoulders and hip using either the handles or gripping the top slide sheet (see fig. 112 on the next page)
▶ Hold your hand/s in front of you with relaxed shoulder and elbow;
▶ Ensure the slide sheet is taut before you move;

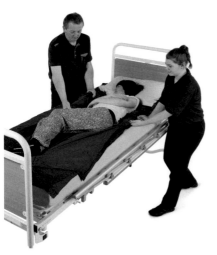

Fig 112

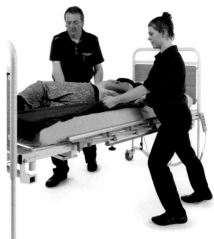

Fig 113

➡ Nominate the handler who will give the commands (the 'lead handler');

➡ The lead handler says clearly 'Ready, steady, slide';

➡ On the command 'slide' the handlers transfer their body weight from front foot (see fig. 113) to back foot (see fig. 114) leaning their weight to execute the move and not pulling using the arms alone;

➡ Make sure the move is controlled, smooth and gentle, and not jerky and/or fast;

➡ If necessary repeat the move until the individual is in the required position (several small moves are preferable to one long move);

➡ Ensure the individual is safe and comfortable, and use correctly fitted safe sides if necessary;

➡ Remove the slide sheet, or if you are using a bed system leave this in place.

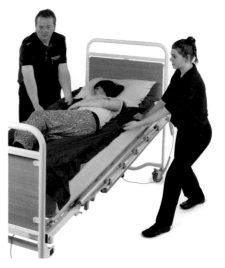

Fig 114

Assisting as a single carer

➡ Generally when a single carer is working alone, the individual to be moved should be lying on an in-situ, sliding bed system rather than by execution of the move using inserted sliding sheets. The carer should proceed as follows;

➡ Raise a safe side on the opposite side of the bed;

➡ Stand at the head end of the bed (the handler can stand behind the pillow at the top of the bed if there is no headboard);

➡ Face the opposite bottom corner of the bed (the oblique position) (see fig. 115)

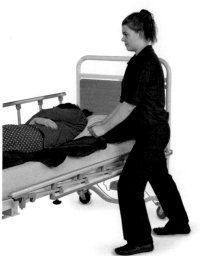

Fig 115

➡ Adopt the basic, base walk-stance of feet slightly apart and one foot in advance of the other;

➡ Hold the top layer of slide sheet by the individual's shoulder or shoulder and hip using either the handles or gripping the top slide sheet (see fig. 116)

➡ Hold your hand/s in front of you with relaxed shoulder and elbow;

➡ Ensure the slide sheet is taut before you move;

➡ As you slide the sheet, transfer your body weight from front foot (see fig. 116) to back foot (see fig. 117) leaning your weight to execute the move and not pulling using your arms alone;

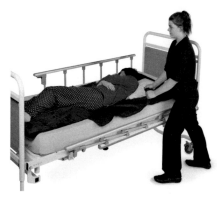

Fig 116

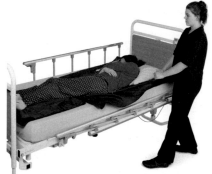

Fig 117

➡ Make sure the move is controlled, smooth and gentle, and not jerky and/or fast;

➡ If necessary, repeat the move until the individual is in the required position (several small moves are preferable to one long move);

➡ As when working from one side of the bed, the individual will have moved up and across the bed, you must go to the other side of the bed and repeat the move to centre the individual;

➡ Ensure the individual is safe and comfortable; use correctly fitted safe sides if necessary;

➡ Remove the slide sheet, or if you are using a bed system leave this in place.

Repositioning Into The Centre Of The Bed

When an individual is turned on to his or her side in the bed, he or she will end up close to the edge of the bed and will need to be repositioned towards the centre. This is best achieved with a slide sheet as it reduces friction and the effort necessary whilst protecting tissue viability.

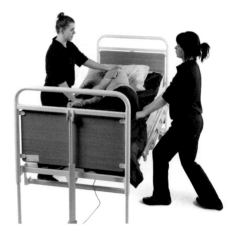

This method can also be used to move the individual closer to the edge during personal care thus reducing the distance a carer must reach across the bed (see fig. 118)

Fig. 118

Assist as follows

➡ Carers stand on each side of the bed, or a single carer raises a bed rail on the opposite side of the bed for safety;

➡ Insert the slide sheet under the individual between all points of contact and the bed surface. If the individual can move his or her own head and feet then the slide sheet can be inserted just under the shoulders and hips;

➡ Get the individual to lie on his or her back until he or she is moved across the bed;

➡ One carer stands at the side of the bed, adopting the basic, walk stance, facing across the bed;

➡ Holding the top layer of the slide sheet close to the bed and at the individual's shoulder and hip (see fig. 119) the carer transfers his or her weight from the front foot on to their back foot, drawing the individual across the bed (see fig. 120)

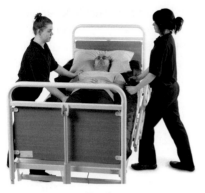 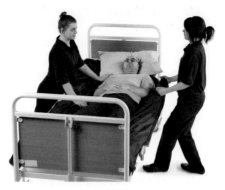

Fig.119   *Fig.120*

- Ask the individual to face the direction in which he or she is turning with his or her arm across the body and a leg bent ready to turn (see fig. 121)
- Stand again with weight on the front foot, holding the slide sheet with hands slightly raised from the bed (do not lift the individual) and again transfer weight on to the back foot (see fig. 122)
- The slide sheet will facilitate the turn, but in some instances it will help if the second carer assists the individual to roll on to his or her side;
- Consider further adjustment of the hips as this may leave the individual in a better position on the bed; if executing this move, use the same action of transferring body weight but this time hold the slide sheet close to the individual's hip;
- Ensure the individual is in a safe position in the bed and if he or she is not, adjust by repeating the slide manoeuvre;
- Remove the slide sheet;
- Review the success of the manoeuvre and reassess as necessary.

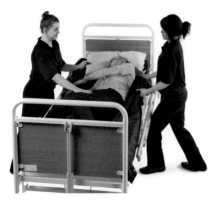 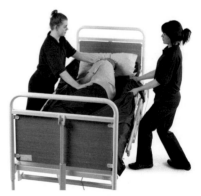

Fig.121   *Fig.122*

Lateral Transfer

There are now devices which can execute a lateral transfer mechanically, thus eliminating the need for a manual handling technique. However, if these are not available then the same technique as for sliding up the bed and repositioning can be used for lateral transfer.

There are a wide range of assistive devices which can execute lateral transfer, but in any case the stance and action required will be as described below. The aid/aids used must ensure that any gap is bridged with a supporting surface (e.g., a transfer board) and that the move can be executed with the friction reduction of a slide system. Single-use slide sheets, specifically designed for lateral transfer, are now available (see following photographs).

Assist as follows:

- ➡ Insert the sliding sheet under the individual;
- ➡ Introduce the transfer board under the individual between the slide sheet and the bed (the individual's head must be on the board and sufficient board available to 'bridge' any gap);
- ➡ Turn the individual on to his or her back (usually a pillow should be used to support the neck and head);
- ➡ Bring the destination surface close to the bed and ensure all brakes are on;
- ➡ Ensure that the destination surface is slightly lower than the surface the individual is leaving;
- ➡ Identify the number of carers required (assessment of every situation is required, but commonly a minimum of three carers (and sometimes more) will be needed for high dependency situations where the head and/or feet of the individual need support);
- ➡ All the carers adopt the basic stance:
  - ➡ If pushing start with weight on the back foot;
  - ➡ If pulling take hold of the slide sheet at appropriate points to control the whole body of the individual and start with the weight on the front foot (see fig. 123)
- ➡ Nominate one carer to lead the move and give the command 'Ready, steady, slide';
- ➡ All carers transfer their weight in the direction of the movement, bringing the individual to the edge of the bed (see fig. 124)

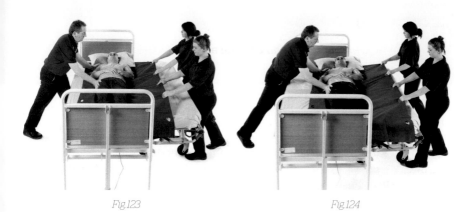

Fig.123   Fig.124

➡ All carers move back into the start position and regather the slide sheet (see fig.125)
➡ Repeat the move to bring the individual across and on to the destination surface
(the carer pushing will stop before he or she overreaches) (see fig. 126)
➡ Remove the transfer aids and ensure the individual is safe and comfortable.

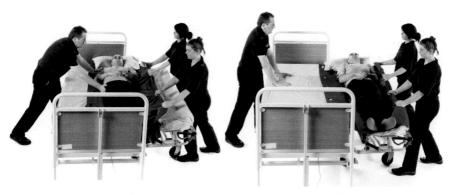

Fig.125   Fig.126

Unit 16
Encouraging Independent Mobility

Wherever possible an individual should be encouraged to complete any move independently. In order to make this easier, the individual should follow the normal movement patterns for the actions described below, so long as they do not have physical limitations which prevent this.

Moving forward in a chair

The individual should:

- ➡ Lean forward in the chair;
- ➡ Lean over to one side and place their weight on one buttock (see fig. 127)
- ➡ Then lift the other buttock clear of the seat and hitch the hip forward as the knee comes across (see fig. 128)
- ➡ Repeat the movement with the other hip (see fig. 129)

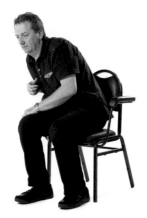
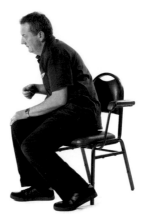
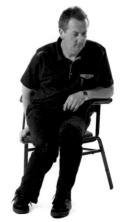

Fig.127   Fig.128   Fig.129

Moving back in a chair

The individual should:

➡ Lean forward in the chair;
➡ Then lean over to one side to place the weight on one buttock;
➡ Lift the other buttock clear of the seat and hitch the hip backward;
➡ Repeat the movement with the other hip.

Standing

The individual should:

➡ Position themselves with their feet flat on the floor and with a stable base (commonly, feet astride and one foot slightly under the body). The individual may need to shuffle forward on the chair or bed in order to achieve this;
➡ Then, looking ahead and pushing with the arms, either from the mattress or the chair arms, the individual should lead with the head and move forward and up into a standing position (see fig. 130 and fig. 131)

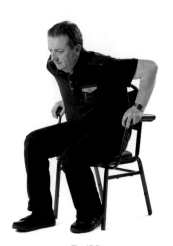

Fig 130

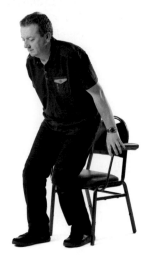

Fig 131

Some individuals benefit from rocking slightly back and forth before attempting to stand up, and if a person has difficulty standing from a chair or bed, it would be worth considering the benefits of raising the furniture to a more suitable height.

Sitting

The individual should:

▸ Stand close to the chair or bed and be able to feel the edge with the back of the legs;
▸ Then reach back and down to position the individual with his or her bottom leading the move (see fig. 132)
▸ Keep the head over the feet (e.g. looking at the feet) enabling him or her to control the speed of descent during the move.

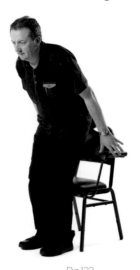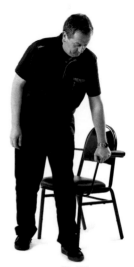

Fig.132   Fig.133

Some individuals find it easier to look at the chair and reach down with one hand in order to sit (see fig. 133)

Getting into bed

▸ Ensure the height of the bed is appropriate for the individual to sit on the side of the bed with the feet firmly on the floor (the lower the height, the easier it is to sit well on to the bed);
▸ If a profile back rest is available, raise it for the individual to lean against;
▸ Sit the individual far enough up the bed to prevent the need for repositioning once the individual is in the bed;

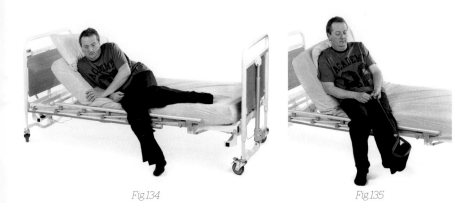

Fig. 134   Fig. 135

→ Side lie the individual, propped on the elbow, and raise legs one at a time on to the bed (see fig. 134)
→ Once the individual is on the bed, roll over or 'bridge' to achieve the right position.

OR

→ If the individual feels able and the edge of the bed is firm, ask him or her to sit at an oblique angle to the bed, lean back on to the pillows or back rest, lift the legs on to the bed and shuffle or 'bridge' to move across the bed (see fig. 135)

Aids which will help:

→ **Bed rail** (see fig. 136)
→ **Bed sheet with satinised panel to aid movement in bed** (see fig. 137)
→ **Rope ladder** (see fig. 138 on the next page)
→ **Hand blocks** (see fig. 139 on the next page)
→ **Profile bed.**

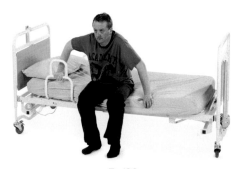

Fig. 136

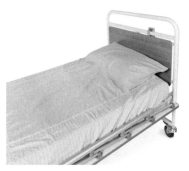

Fig. 137

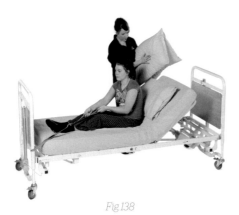

Fig.138

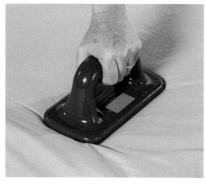

Fig.139

Getting out of bed

➡ Ask the individual to turn on to his or her side (or assist him or her in rolling) (see fig. 140)
➡ Ask the individual to draw the knees up and towards the edge of the bed (this will allow the legs to drop over the edge of the bed naturally as the individual sits up) (see fig. 141)
➡ Get the individual to place the upper hand on to the bed and push up on to the elbow;
➡ Ask the individual to slide his or her feet over the edge of the bed (a slide sheet under the feet will facilitate this, but do not let it fall to the floor where it would become a tripping or slipping hazard);
➡ As the feet come off the side of the bed, get the individual to push up against the bed or grab rail to bring him or her into a sitting position (see fig. 142)

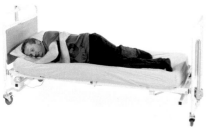

Fig.140

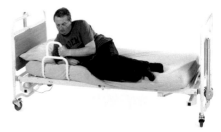

Fig.141

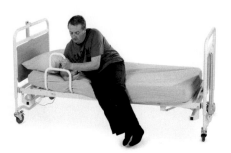

Fig 142

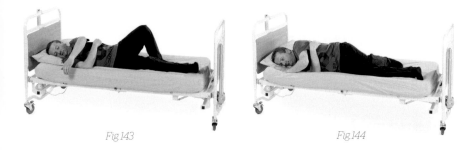

Fig 143   Fig 144

Rolling in bed

Many individuals can turn on to their side if encouraged to. Get them to:

- Look in the direction of the turn;
- Raise the far leg and place the foot against the mattress;
- Push with this foot as he or she reaches across the body in the direction of the turn (see fig. 143 and fig. 144)

Some individuals can turn by pulling themselves over using a bed rail designed for the purpose (however, pulling on 'cot sides' is not recommended).

Note: Pulling to roll alters the normal movement action for turning: grasping the lever, the person uses a PULLING (flexion) pattern for the upper body instead of REACHING (extension) in the direction of motion. It is harder to pull when pushing through the foot, so individuals will tend to just use the upper body to pull themselves over.

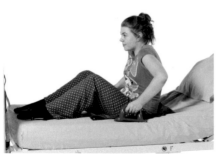 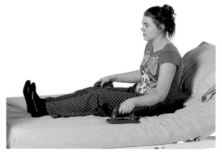

Fig.145   Fig.146

Moving up the bed

By providing an individual with small handling aids such as hand blocks and small slide sheets he or she may be able to move up the bed (see fig. 145 and fig. 146).

Sitting up in bed

Using a rope ladder may enable an individual to support his or her own sitting position, as a carer positions pillows (see fig. 147)

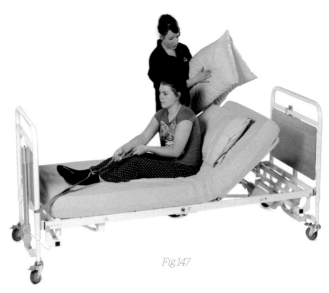

Fig.147

Unit 17
Methods of Assistance

Methods of Assisting People

The following methods of assisting people are ways, if necessary, to facilitate movement and assist an individual to change position or move from one place to the next. The methods described are not the only ways to move individuals but form a set of core techniques which will be suitable for many situations. It is beyond the scope of a single publication to describe all the possible and suitable methods, and by referring to specific publications on moving and handling, you will develop your knowledge and understanding of other practices.

Always encourage individuals to move independently wherever possible, even if they can only help with part of the move.

Only assist individuals where it is required and then only to the level required as this will encourage individuals to do some of the moving themselves.

Before assisting an individual with any move, ensure you have read his or her moving and handling plan, which will inform you of what equipment should be used, the number of carers required and any other specific, relevant information regarding the individual.

If equipment is to be used, ensure it is the correct item and the right size; check it for safety and cleanliness; and make sure you are trained in how to use it.

Report any faulty equipment and do not use.

Before commencing any of the methods described below, make sure you have read and are using the information from the chapters on:

▶ Basic Stance;
▶ Standard Preparation;
▶ General use of Equipment.

The points from these chapters will not be reiterated for each method but do still need to be applied.

Assist Forward and Back in the Chair

If assistance is required, then proceed as follows:

- Create a stable base using a half kneel position in front of the individual;
- Ask the individual to lean forward and across to one side so that his or her weight is on one buttock;
- Place an open hand on the hip of the raised buttock;
- Rest the other hand at the knee (see fig. 148)
- On the command of 'shuffle' ease the individual's hip across and towards the front of the chair thus facilitating forward movement of the thigh, with the knee coming across to facilitate the move (see fig. 149) transfer your weight back as you do this so as not to pull with your arms;
- Repeat this sequence with the other leg (see fig. 150)
- Ensure the individual is balanced and safe in the final sitting position;
- Ensure the individual's feet are firmly placed on the floor.

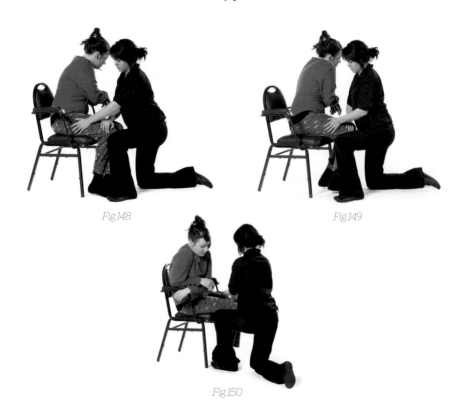

Fig 148   Fig 149

Fig 150

To shuffle back in the chair reverse the process

If assistance is required consider seating the individual on a one-way glide sheet and using a pillow in front of the individual's knees (this can protect him or her from excessive pressure or bruising), then proceed as follows:

- ⊡ Kneel in front of the individual with one leg raised (half kneeling) to create a stable base;
- ⊡ Ask the individual to lean his or her weight forward and to one side;
- ⊡ Place an open hand at the hip or on the thigh of the individual on the side he or she has lifted off the seat;

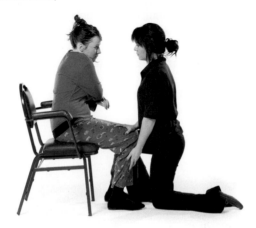

Fig 151

- ⊡ Rest the other hand below the knee (see fig. 151)
- ⊡ On the command of 'shuffle' transfer your weight forward while also gently pushing the individual back in the chair as he or she hitches back;
- ⊡ Then get the individual to lean over towards alternate sides and the move is repeated;
- ⊡ If the individual is sitting on a one-way glide sheet, rest a hand below each knee and gently push the individual back;
- ⊡ Ensure the individual is balanced and safe in the final sitting position;
- ⊡ Ensure the feet are firmly placed on the floor.

If the individual needs repeated assistance to sit up in the chair then review his or her assessment and consider the factors that could be making him or her slump in the chair. Consider, for example, the effects of excessive fatigue or whether the design of the chair is incorrect for the individual or whether the individual is being left sitting in the chair for an inappropriate duration.

Assist To Stand

If assistance is required then proceed as follows:

- ➡ Ensure the individual is wearing appropriate footwear;
- ➡ If the individual is able to push, ask him or her to place their hands on the arms of the chair or the mattress;
- ➡ Then ask the individual to look ahead;
- ➡ Check that the individual is able to sit upright unsupported and can raise his or her feet from or lower his or her feet to the floor; if the individual cannot, report the situation or assist with caution;
- ➡ Stand beside the individual facing the direction of movement (see fig. 152)
- ➡ Adopt the basic walk stance with the outer foot ahead;
- ➡ Adjust height by flexing at the hips and knees;
- ➡ Place your hand on the central key point to prompt a standing movement (see fig. 153)
- ➡ Stabilise the individual at the end of the move and proceed with a walk.

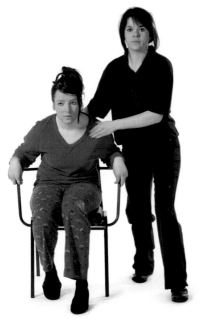

Fig 152

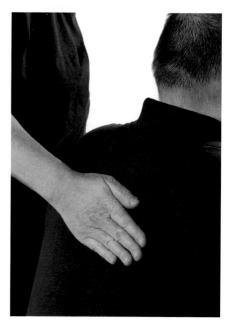

Fig 153

OR for a less able individual:

➡ Place your inside forearm in contact with the individual's back (a 'long arm hold'; if the individual is on a bed, turning him or her slightly in one direction gives access for a long arm hold) (see fig. 154 and fig. 155)

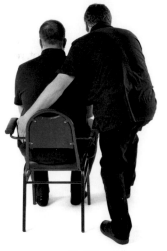
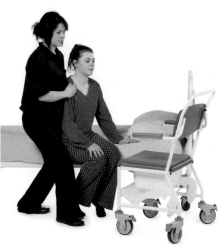

Fig 154   *Fig 155*

➡ Support the individual with your outer hand either at the individual's shoulder or with a palm to palm hold (see fig. 156)
➡ Look ahead;
➡ Say clearly 'Ready, steady, stand' (a gentle rocking motion can be used as the commands are given);
➡ On the command 'stand' both move together in the direction of movement, travelling forward and then upwards (see fig. 157 on the next page)
➡ Transfer your body weight from the back foot to the front foot or step forward with the back foot;
➡ If the individual is unsteady, ask them to sit down or transfer him or her to another sitting point (see fig. 158 on the next page)

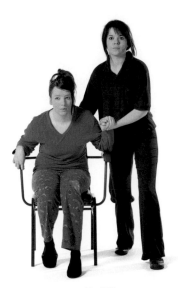

Fig 156

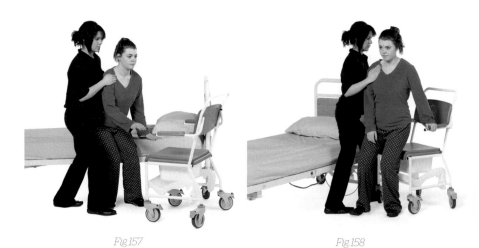

Fig 157   *Fig 158*

Alternatively

➡ Support the individual with a front oblique hold by standing to one side of the individual and transferring your weight from the front foot to the back foot (see fig. 159)

Note:

➡ The carer may need to change direction in order to progress to a walk, which could make the individual unbalanced;
➡ The carer must not stand directly in front of the individual as this will block movement and the individual could pull on the carer.

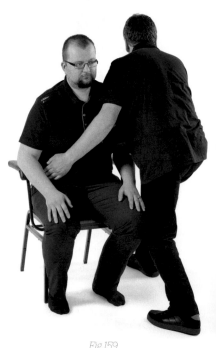

Fig 159

Assist to Walk and Sit

Ideally the individual will be walking independently or using an aid and the handler will be giving verbal or touch-prompt guidance only.

If an individual needs extra support to maintain a standing position, he or she should be provided with an aid such as a walking frame or stick.

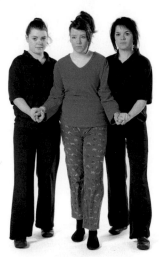
Fig.160

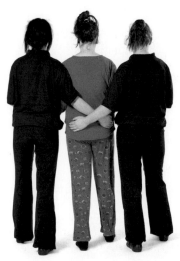
Fig.161

Assessments should identify how many handlers will be required, but if the individual is unsteady or unpredictable when walking two handlers (see fig. 160 and fig. 161) are preferable for optimum support, and it may be advisable to follow the individual with a wheelchair so he or she can sit down if necessary (see fig. 162)

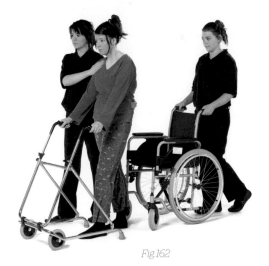
Fig.162

If assistance is required then proceed as follows:

➡ Assess how far the individual is able to walk before needing to sit down (it may be beneficial to have a chair ready at a half way stage);

➡ If necessary, ensure the individual has any aid required such as a walking frame

(Note: handlers must not rest a foot on a walking frame to steady it or allow the individual to pull up on it: the individual should always stand first and then take hold of the frame);

➡ If the individual is using a walking aid such as a stick, make sure it is held in the opposite hand to any injury (e.g. right hand following left hip surgery) and you should walk on the opposite side (the individual's weaker side);

➡ Make sure you are present and guiding but do not give substantial support to maintain a standing position. If the individual leans continuously on you then stop the walk, sit the individual down in a wheelchair and continue the transfer by this means;

➡ To guide the individual, place your near arm across the individual's lower back, flat palm in centre or at far pelvis;

➡ Support at the shoulder or nearside ribs (see fig. 163 and fig. 164)

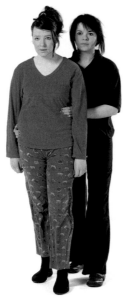
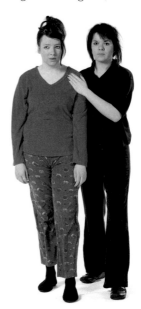

Fig 163

Fig 164

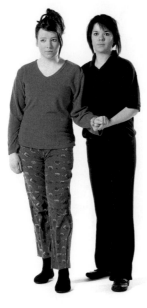 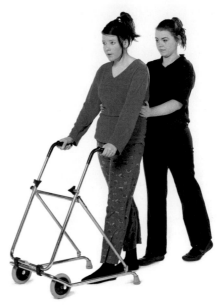

Fig.165   *Fig.166*

Alternatively, if the individual needs guiding:

➡ Take a palm to palm hold (see fig. 165), but do not link thumbs, holding at about hip height, and not higher than waist height;
➡ Do not let the individual push down on your guiding hand; if the individual does, stop, release the hold, take a shoulder or rib support and continue. If the individual is able to push down he or she might benefit from a walking aid;
➡ Adopt a stable base with feet slightly apart and the outer foot ahead, ready to step with the person;
➡ Keep as close to the individual as necessary (usually slightly behind them with your hip close to the individual's pelvis);
➡ Do not impede the individual's natural step or his or her walking aid;
➡ Allow the individual to move his or her feet in his or her own time;
➡ If the individual uses a walking frame then you can help the individual with his or her confidence and balance by walking behind, but slightly to one side to ensure clear vision, placing your hands just above the individual's hips (see fig. 166)

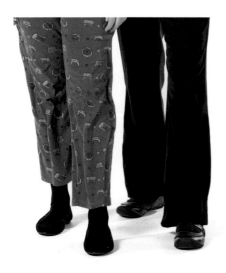 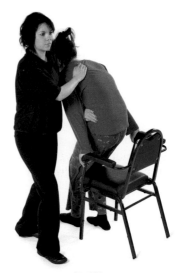

Fig 167   *Fig 168*

➡ Unison walking (i.e. stepping with the same foot as the individual) can be helpful for some individuals (e.g. those with dementia (see fig. 167)

➡ On arriving at the destination, ensure the individual can see the chair and ask him or her to reach for an arm of it as he or she turns and to sit, leading with the bottom;

➡ If an individual requires additional assistance:

   ➡ Let him or her turn until the back of the legs are in contact with the chair;

   ➡ Ask the individual to reach down with both hands;

   ➡ Steady the individual by stepping in the direction he or she is sitting;

   ➡ Guide the individual's hip back towards the chair but keep the shoulder inclining forward (see fig. 168)

Use Of A Sitting Transfer Board

This move is predominantly an independent transfer: the handler is present for preparation and completion but gives minimal assistance during the actual transfer.

Note: If a curved board is used it is safest to have the short edge next to the individual's knees so that he or she travels along the short edge. The long edge is thus supported and the board is less likely to tip.

Once you have ensured that the individual feels able to undertake the activity, encourage him or her to move as follows:

- Place the feet flat on the floor or on a turn disc if required (placing a turn disc under the individual's feet can be beneficial as it allows the feet to follow through as the individual transfers);
- Place the board under one buttock (see fig. 169) and ensure it is safely on the destination surface (do not have more than one third of the board unsupported across a gap);
- Ask the individual to place his or her hand towards the far end of the board and to lean in the same direction (see fig. 170)

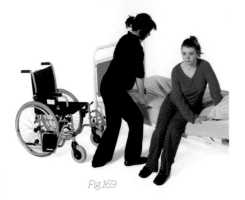

Fig 169

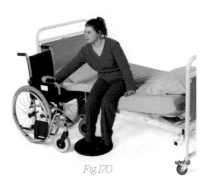

Fig 170

- When the individual is ready ask him or her to shuffle across, using the hands to push (the individual should have his or her feet in contact with the floor and push through the feet if he or she is able to do it);
- Get the individual to transfer his or her weight in the direction of the move;
- The individual eases the hips across the board (see fig. 171)

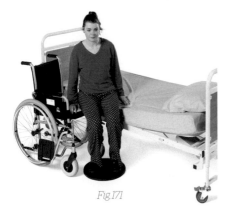

Fig 171

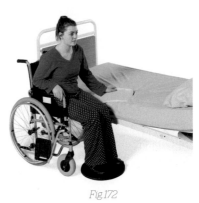

Fig 172

➡ Ensure the individual is safely on the receiving point (see fig. 172)

➡ Then remove the board, asking the individual to lean or rock away from the board to facilitate the removal (if in use, remove turn disc from under the feet);

➡ If a wheelchair was used and the arm of the wheelchair was removed before the transfer, replace the arm of the wheelchair; also ensure the individual's feet are on the wheelchair footplates.

If the individual requires additional assistance then:

➡ Establish a stable base half-kneeling in front of the individual;

➡ Place a hand on the individual's hip furthest from the receiving point and help initiate the move (the individual should not be pushed across (see fig. 173)

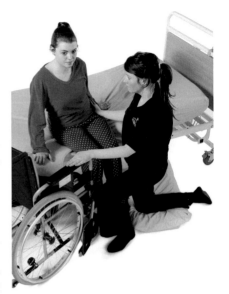

Fig 173

Note: If significant physical effort is required to assist the individual an alternative method should be considered (e.g. hoisting).

Use Of A Standing Transport Aid

Assist as follows:

➡ Check that the handle height and shin pad (if adjustable) are adjusted to the correct height for the individual (see the handling plan);

➡ Ensure the individual can comprehend and follow instruction and can lift his or her feet off the floor;

➡ Ensure the individual is wearing suitable footwear;

➡ Where possible ask the individual to move to the front of the chair in readiness to stand;

➡ Place the transporter directly in front of the individual;

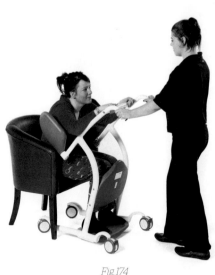
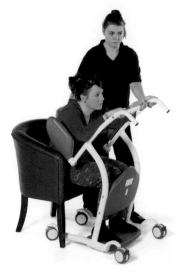

Fig.174   *Fig.175*

➡ Apply the brakes;

➡ Ask the individual to place his or her feet on to the footplate;

➡ Ask the individual to move slightly forward in the chair until his or her shins are against the pad (see fig. 174)

➡ Stand facing the individual and hold the handles;

➡ Ask the individual to place his or her hands on the handle bar and to pull up into a standing position (if an individual has difficulty with this, a carer can assist) (see fig. 175)

➡ Encourage the individual to remain in an upright position as the seat is brought into position;

➡ Ask the individual to hold on as he or she sits back on to the seat;

➡ Remove the brakes and reassure the individual during the transfer, and transport short distances only (see fig. 176 on the next page)

➡ At the destination apply the brakes;

➡ Ask the individual to come up into a standing position;

➡ Remove the seat and ask the individual to sit down (if the individual has difficulty with this, a carer can assist);

➡ Ask the individual to lift his or her feet off the transporter and remove the transporter carefully;

➡ Ensure the individual is safe and comfortable, encouraging him or her to shuffle back in the chair if necessary.

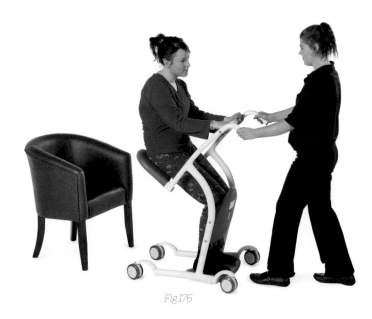

Fig. 176

Assistance to Sit up in Bed

Use of profile beds that bring an individual into a sitting position (see fig. 177) remove the need for manual assistance of an individual into a sitting position. Profile beds have been found to improve tissue viability and also increase an individual's independence as he or she may well be able to use the profile function without assistance.

Alternatively, a pillow lifter could be used for the same purpose.

If assistance is required proceed as follows:

➡ Start in the basic walk stance in an oblique position to the bed and facing the individual (see fig. 178)

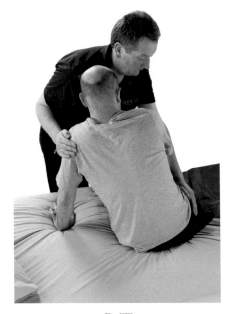

Fig. 177

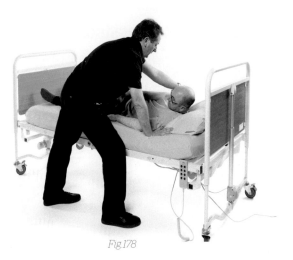

Fig.178

➡ Flex at the hips and knees;

➡ Ask the individual to raise his or her head off the bed and at the same time guide the shoulder across and down the bed until the individual is resting on the elbow. At the same time transfer your body weight from the front to the back foot (see fig.179)

➡ Ask the individual to push up to a sitting position and to support him/herself by bending one knee and placing the hand/s behind the body as a prop on the bed (see fig. 180)

➡ Adjust the pillows;

➡ Ensure the individual is safe and comfortable (use correctly fitted safe sides/bed rails if required).

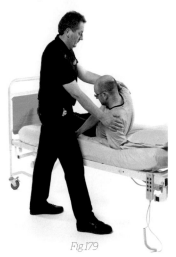

Fig 179

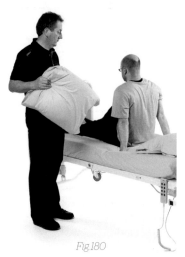

Fig 180

Alternative methods of assistance

1. The individual may be able to use a rope ladder fixed from the end of the bed in order to pull him/herself up into a sitting position (see fig. 181)

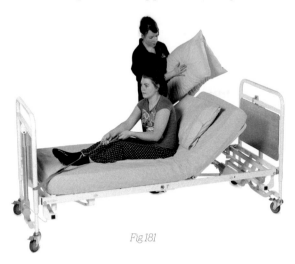

Fig.181

2. Two handlers can assist an individual into a sitting position in the following manner when a profile bed is unavailable (however, a profile bed should be provided where possible):

⮞ Place a handling strap behind the individual's shoulders (see fig. 182)

⮞ Standing on either side of the bed each adopt the basic stance, flexing and placing your weight on the foot nearest the head of the bed (see fig. 183)

⮞ Hold the strap with the inside hand;

⮞ Make sure the individual can bring his or her chin towards the chest when he or she is sitting to prevent the head falling back;

⮞ Get the individual to bend the knees slightly;

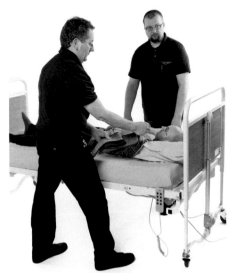

Fig.182

➡ On the command 'ready, steady, sit' transfer your weight on to the back foot, bringing the individual up into a sitting position (see fig. 184)

➡ If an additional task is required, such as placing extra pillows, a third carer may be required if the individual cannot support him/herself once sitting.

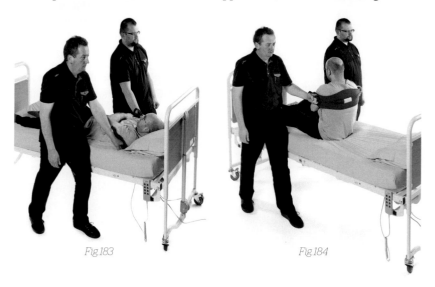

Fig 183   *Fig 184*

Assistance To Get Into Bed

A height adjustable profile bed will assist the transfer. Raise the profile back rest up for the individual to lean into.

If a profile bed is not available then several pillows will prevent the individual falling back as he or she transfers into the bed.

Ensure the height of the bed is appropriate for the individual to sit on the side of the bed with his or her feet firmly on the floor (the lower the bed, the easier it is to sit well on to it).

If the individual feels able and the edge of the bed is firm, ask the individual to sit on the bed at an oblique angle and lie back against the profile bed or pillows and raise the legs one at a time (see fig. 185 on the next page)

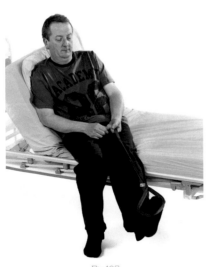

Fig 185

The individual's bottom will create resistance against the bed sheet as the legs are transferred into the bed and this will have an impact on tissue viability and is thus undesirable; it also makes the legs feel heavier to the handler. This can be prevented by sitting the individual on equipment designed to reduce friction such as:

→ A satinised base sheet on the bed (see chapter on Encouraging Independent Mobility);
→ A turn disc;
→ A slide sheet with a non-slip edge;
→ A slide sheet with handles designed to be held during the manoeuvre to prevent the individual slipping off the bed.

Caution: using a standard slide sheet under the bottom will reduce the friction, but if the individual's legs are lifted across into the centre of the bed the hip is likely to move to the edge of the bed and the individual could fall to the floor.

A small roller slide sheet or folded flat sheet on the foot of the bed for the ankles and calves makes it easier to position the individual's legs without lifting.

If assistance is required proceed as follows:

→ Position the back rest of the profile bed at approximately 45° (or place pillows ready for the individual to lean into);
→ If necessary place a slide sheet at the foot end of the bed;
→ Ask the individual to sit as far on to the bed as he or she can and lean on to or side lie on the profile backrest or the pillows;

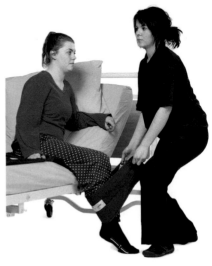

Fig 186

- ➡ Place a handling strap behind the individual's lower calf;
- ➡ Position yourself facing the foot of the bed with the individual's legs in front of you (see fig. 186)
- ➡ Start from a power squat and raise the legs by coming up into a standing position (see fig. 187)
- ➡ Walk towards the bed and position the legs on to the side of the bed (see fig. 188)
- ➡ Slide the legs into the bed until they are comfortable and remove the slide sheet from under them and the turn disc from under the hips (see fig. 189)
- ➡ Once the individual has rolled on to his or her back he or she can then shuffle into a comfortable position.

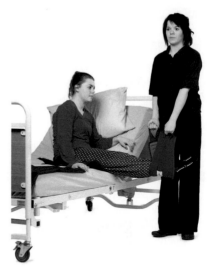

Fig 187

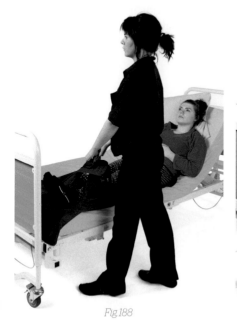

Fig 188

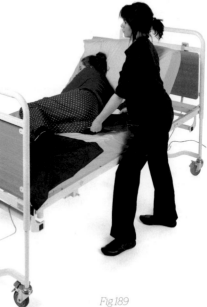

Fig 189

Assistance to Get Out of Bed

If assistance is required proceed as follows:

▪ Ask the individual to turn on to his or her side or assist the individual to roll (see below, rolling an individual in bed);

▪ Ask or assist the individual to draw the knees up and towards the edge of the bed (see fig. 190) (this will allow the legs to drop over the edge of the bed naturally as the individual sits);

▪ Adopt the basic stance with an oblique position to the top end of the bed and close to the individual;

▪ Ask the individual to push up on to the elbow or assist him or her to do this by placing a hand under the shoulder (see fig. 191 and fig. 192) and transfer your weight on to your back foot as you assist;

▪ Ask the individual to draw his or her knees up and slide the feet over the edge of the bed or assist the individual to do this (a slide sheet under the feet facilitates this (see fig. 193));

▪ As the feet come off the side of the bed, the individual should push up against the bed to bring him/herself into a sitting position;

▪ If the individual needs assistance, adopt an oblique stance towards the bottom of the bed and place a hand at the shoulder and a hand on the hip (see fig. 194) and transfer your weight on to your front foot as the individual pushes up (see fig. 195)

▪ Support the individual (see fig. 196) or ask him or her to support him/herself as the bed is lowered until the feet are on the ground.

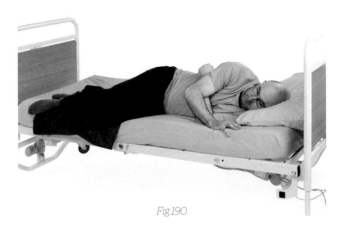

Fig 190

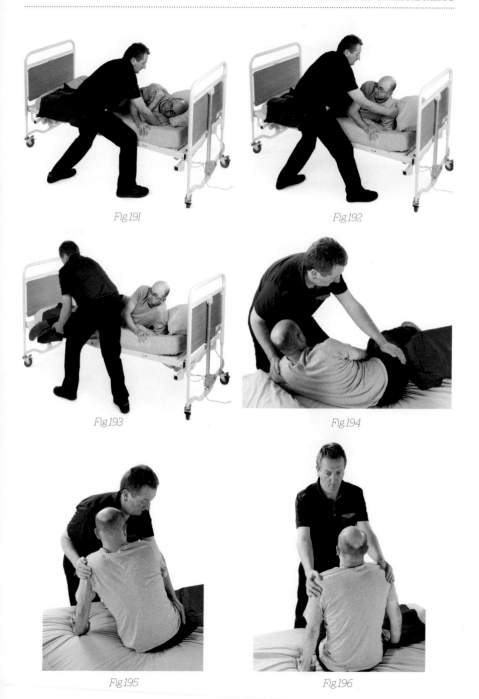

Fig 191

Fig 192

Fig 193

Fig 194

Fig 195

Fig 196

Rolling an Individual in Bed

If assistance is required proceed as follows:

▶ Ask the individual to look in the direction of the turn, reach across with his or her arm and bend the knee of the far leg;

▶ Ensure the arm on the side the individual is turning towards is away from the body creating a space;

▶ Stand at the side of the bed the individual is to face and adopt the basic stance;

▶ Place an open palm hold on the individual's shoulder blade and pelvis or knee, but do not grip (see fig. 197)

▶ Say clearly 'Ready, steady, roll';

▶ On the command 'roll', transfer your body weight from your front foot on to the back foot;

▶ Assist the individual to roll, ideally letting the individual's shoulder lead the move;

▶ Move back in towards the side of the bed and stand close to it (see fig. 198)

▶ A second handler can assist by pushing at the same time using the same contact points (see fig. 199) and, from a basic stance, transferring his or her weight from the back foot to the front foot as he or she pushes;

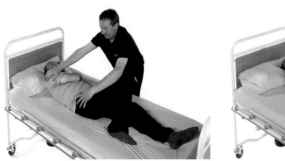

Fig 197   Fig 198

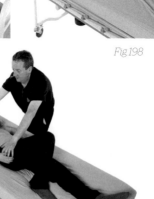

Fig 199

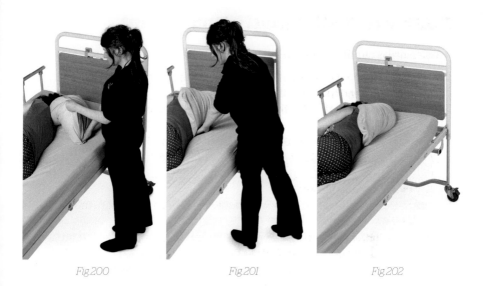

Fig.200   Fig.201   Fig.202

➡ Ensure the individual is safe: use a correctly fitted safe side if necessary;

➡ Ensure the individual is comfortable, inserting additional pillows if necessary;

➡ A pillow can be used to support side lying, removing the need for a carer to hold the individual during personal care . To remove the need for a carer to hold the individual, support side lying by:

> ➡ Getting the individual to put his or her face on one corner of a pillow and then take the opposite corner and twist the pillow (see fig. 200)

> ➡ Push the twisted corner under the individual's shoulder (see fig. 201)

> ➡ Ask the individual to lean back into the pillow (see fig. 202)

> Note: In a very high dependency situation, additional handlers will be required to support at additional points so that the individual's whole body is rolled in unison in, for example, a log roll.

If the individual needs to be repositioned centrally in the bed, then insert and use the slide sheet as described in the chapter Use of Slide Sheets.

Falls: Prevention And Management

The risk factors involved in falls can be divided into three main groups:

1. Intrinsic – medical, physical and functional ability of the individual.
2. Extrinsic – environmental factors.
3. Behavioural – mental health and cognitive level of the individual.

(Masud & Morris 2001 - Steinhoef et al 2002)

The management of falls should be based on identifying the contributory factors and taking action to reduce the likelihood of the individual falling.

Organisations should ensure they have a falls strategy or policy and that they investigate any falls. Individuals at risk from falls should have a specific falls and manual handling assessment. This assessment should take account of any factor that is likely to have an impact on the likelihood of the individual falling or not (e.g. medication, poor lighting at night or an unfamiliar environment).

Assistive technology can be used to reduce the likelihood of falls: for example, sensors can be placed on chairs, beds or floors, or even around the whole room, to alert a carer to the fact that the individual is up and moving.

Environments should be assessed to ensure the risks created are reduced to as low a level as is reasonably practicable.

Assisting Someone Up From The Floor

If you come across an individual on the floor, ensure he or she is not hurt or injured and reassure him or her. If you are in any doubt, call for medical assistance.

Then follow your organisation's procedures and the individual's manual handling plan.

If the individual is unable to move then equipment such as a raising cushion or a hoist will be required.

If assistance is required proceed as follows:

➡ Ensure there is sufficient space around the individual;
➡ Bring a suitable chair close to the individual, so that he or she can push up on it;
➡ A second chair or stool can also be brought for the individual to sit back on;

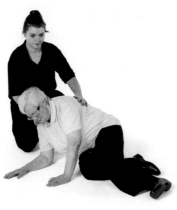 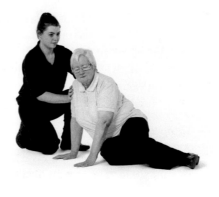

Fig.203   Fig.204

➡ Kneel on the floor beside the individual, adopting a position which allows appropriate flexion and spinal alignment and a stable base, or sit on a chair beside the individual;

➡ Avoid stooping over the individual;

➡ Bring the chair/s close to the individual;

➡ Ask or assist the individual to roll on to his or her side, bend both knees with the outer leg over the leg on the floor, raise up on to an elbow and push up with the other hand until in a side sitting position (see fig. 203 and fig. 204)

➡ Ask or assist the individual to turn on to his or her hands and knees (see fig. 205)

➡ Place a chair so the individual can lean his or her hands on the seat of the chair (see fig. 206)

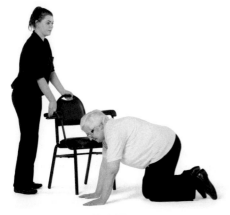 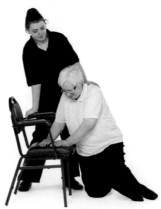

Fig.205   Fig.206

- ➡ Ask the individual to raise a knee and place the foot on the floor (this can be easier to achieve if the individual leans over one knee before attempting to lift the other leg through (see fig. 207));
- ➡ A second chair can be placed behind or slightly to one side of the individual (see fig. 208)
- ➡ Encourage the individual to then push up, turn and sit on the chair or push back on to another chair set behind him or her;
- ➡ The individual should remain seated until he or she has regained his or her balance and confidence before standing or transferring to a wheelchair (see fig. 209)

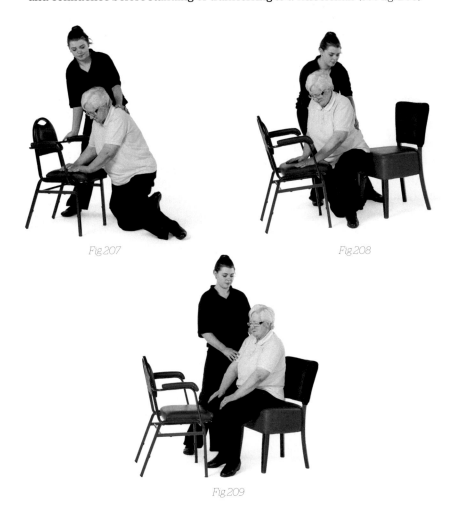

Fig 207   Fig 208

Fig 209

Unit 18
Assisting Babies & Small Children

Children present with a very wide range of needs in relation to moving and handling. Specific methods may be required to meet their needs and these should be devised in discussion with other professionals such as physiotherapists, language therapists, occupational therapists, etc. Any method implemented must take account of not only children's physical needs but also their psychological needs, psycho-social needs, social needs and educational needs. Families must be involved as they will often be providing the continuous, everyday support.

A few basic strategies and methods are described below, but specific training in the moving and handling of children should be given to all who work in child settings. Small children and babies may appear to be in a low risk category for moving and handling but their height and weight are only two aspects which should be considered in a risk assessment. Other aspects may include the likelihood of spasm, low tone, high tone, dystonia, behavioural issues and medical issues, to name but a few.

If children are to be encouraged to reach their full potential in all aspects of their lives it is important that they become as mobile as they possibly can. The moving and handling of children should reflect this desired outcome and therefore should not be unreasonably cautious in involving a child in his or her own movement.

Touch

Children are very sensitive to touch and they gather a lot of information through touch (e.g. children may interpret firm contact as commanding or controlling as well as, or instead of, being merely for the purposes of instruction and support). Tension in the contact hand can give an excessively firm touch and it can be useful to undertake some relaxation exercises before approaching or having physical contact so that any tension in the handler's touch is reduced.

Children don't just use their voices for communication, but all of their senses (touch, sight, hearing, etc). So when you approach a child remember some of the following basic communication skills which can encourage a child to relax, relate and participate such as:

- ▸ 'Open' body language;
- ▸ Gentle, calm and quiet voice tone;
- ▸ Calm, controlled manner of approach;
- ▸ Slow movement as walking quickly will make you talk more quickly and at a higher pitch and volume;
- ▸ Making sure the child is happy for you to commence the move either from the child's verbal cues or from observing the child's body language;
- ▸ Being prepared to wait or even to return in a few minutes;
- ▸ Having a positive expectation: do not invite refusal but expect the child to succeed (e.g. 'We are going to stand now' rather than 'Can you stand up for me');
- ▸ Using positive rather than negative instruction (e.g. 'Stay standing' not 'don't sit down').

> Talking is likely to increase postural tone in children with cerebral palsy: if the child is in a wheelchair and you stand above him or her as you talk he or she will look up, which increases an abnormal extensor pattern of movement.

Touch Cues

Soft and firm touches give different information and both are appropriate for different outcomes, but to give an instruction, try a different type of touch altogether.

For Example:

SOFT: can be used for introduction, to build up confidence and trust;
FIRM: can be used to create a response or action (e.g. to facilitate a standing motion);
INSTRUCTION: can be used to guide, for example, touch the child's hip and then a chair to indicate the instruction, 'sit'.

Facilitation

Using peripheral key points (shoulder and pelvis) to roll:

▶ Increases postural tone in hypotonic children as they activate muscles;

▶ Decreases postural tone in hypertonic children, making it easier for them to move.

The central key point (high central front or back):

▶ Assists in bringing 'nose over toes' to facilitate standing;

▶ Reduces extension when a child is hoisted in a sling.

Lifting aids

Hoists and slings are used for children of all ages and their method of use is the same as for an adult (which is described in the chapter on hoists and slings). Specialist slings such as walking harnesses can be very beneficial when developing standing and walking functions. These slings can also aid complex transfers such as when using specialist standing or walking frames, gym apparatus or even when doing horse riding.

A manual lifting sling is available for children and allows for an interim manual method either for settings where a hoist would not be accessible or as an introduction to slings and future hoisting. The sling is fitted as for a hoist sling but the child is lifted using the handles and following the basic load management principles of:

▶ Identify the number of handlers to be used by undertaking a risk assessment;

▶ Adopt basic stance or power squat if lifting from the floor;

▶ Get a good hold;

▶ Keep the load close;

▶ Keep the transfer distance as short as possible.

Particular care must be taken if the child tends to go into extensor spasm or has unpredictable movement or behaviour patterns.

BABIES

All the principles of basic load management apply when handling small babies along with considerations of how they are moving and responding to touch and whether they have additional special needs.

When transferring babies into seats or buggies (see fig. 210):

- Adopt the basic stance;
- Move your weight over your feet in the direction you are moving the baby;
- Flex in the direction you are moving the baby;
- Keep the baby as close to your body as is possible;
- Give appropriate support to the baby, particularly at the head.

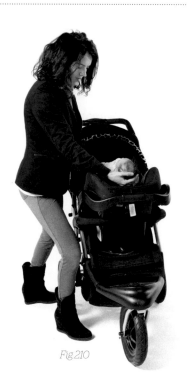

Fig. 210

Variations of holds

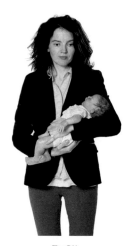

Fig. 211

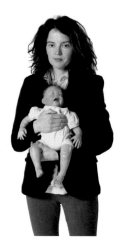

Fig. 212

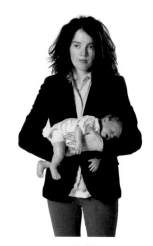

Fig. 213

Small Children

Although it is acceptable to lift small, children a risk assessment must take account of all aspects of the child which could make lifting a significant risk: for example, spasm, unpredictable movement or behaviour, low tone, high tone and handling constraints such as hip spica.

Children respond very differently to strangers and family members or people they know well and this also will impact on the risks of lifting them. It is unwise to make an assumption that it is safe to lift because the child is small.

Variations of holds

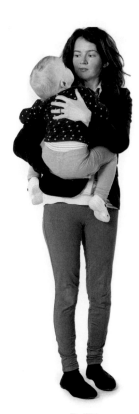

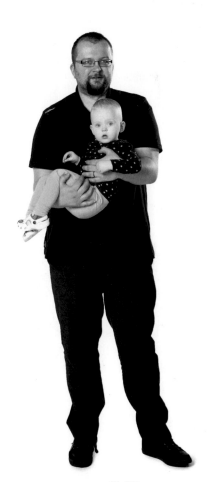

Fig 214   Fig 215

Variations of supporting standing

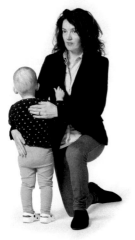 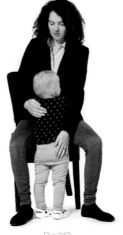 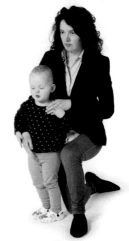

Fig. 216　　　　　　*Fig. 217*　　　　　　*Fig. 218*

Lifting from the floor

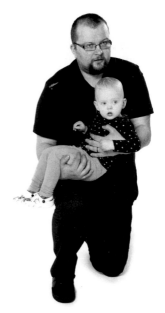

When lifting from or putting down on the floor ensure you have:

- ➡ A stable base;
- ➡ A secure hold;
- ➡ Split the transfer distance where possible (e.g. from chair to floor rather than from standing position to floor).

It may be better to pass the child to a standing person rather than try to stand whilst supporting the child's weight.

Where possible try to support the child's weight through your leg rather than just your arms (see fig. 219).

Fig. 219

Unit 19

Assisting the Person with Dementia

Assisting the Individual with Dementia, Anxiety and Non-Compliant Behaviour

To fully address these issues, carers should receive specialist training.

Always consider how vulnerable you are to harm before you get into a position which could expose you to that harm. For example, kneeling directly in front of a person to apply a sling could expose you to kicking, biting and hitting, whereas standing in a power squat to one side of the person means you can move away more rapidly and are less in the 'direct line of fire'. Obviously, a second person could also support and distract the individual to reduce the likelihood of undesirable reactions.

Individuals with dementia may misinterpret or be confused about familiar features and this can affect their ability to move effectively. For example, a shadow on the floor or a door threshold or a change in the floor surface can all lead to the individual stopping and being reluctant to walk as he or she may be frightened of or be unable to understand what he or she is seeing. Carers need to understand these issues and learn how to avoid or manage them.

Adaptations To Standard Practice

Communication

Identify an appropriate communication method for each individual. Clear, concise instruction and use of goal based communication can be useful (e.g. 'Let us go for a walk' rather than 'Please stand up').

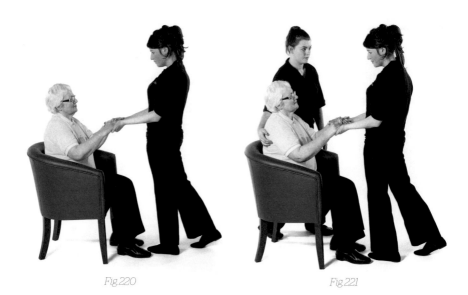

Fig.220   *Fig.221*

SIT TO STAND (gap fill) If the individual is fearful of space then it may help to stand in front of him or her and offer your hands for him or her to take (see fig. 220) Do not pull the individual into a standing position: the individual should stand independently or have a second carer to help him or her stand up (see fig. 221).

Grabbing: keep the individual's hands busy (e.g. with a hankie or stress reliever).

Assisting Walk

(leaning when walking) If the individual leans on you as he or she is walking, stop the walk, reduce direct contact with the individual's body and see if he or she stands better; if not find a chair and sit the individual down for a time as he or she may be tired. The individual may walk better with the help of a walking aid to lean on.

Unison walking: this is stepping with the same foot as the individual (see fig. 222) and helps with walking as he or she is likely to copy your step.

Using a walking frame: the individual may need encouragement to walk into the frame: standing close by and using a touch prompt at the central key point on the back will encourage the individual to walk into the frame. Stand slightly in front of the individual rather than behind as again this encourages the individual to move forward (see fig. 223)

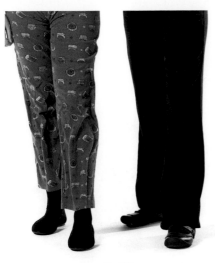 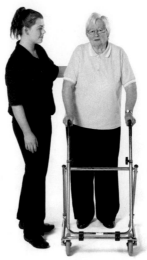

Fig. 222   Fig. 223

Steps and Stairs

Steps and stairs present a significant issue; particularly coming down them. It may be advisable to consider a room downstairs for the individual as stairs are hazardous, with the potential for serious harm should an accident occur. However, some individuals will manage well if they are allowed to face the stair rail, grasp it with both hands and step down sideways, one step at a time.

Chairs

Slumping in the chair can be an indication of illness or tiredness, and that the individual would benefit from a change in position (e.g. a rest on the bed). Slumping may also be an indication that the seating is not appropriate for the individual's needs and a seating assessment should be undertaken.

To sit: allow the individual to keep the chair in sight, walk the individual past the centre of the chair, ask him or her to place his or her hand down on to the arm of the chair and to turn the hips sideways in towards the seat of the chair as the individual sits (see fig. 224 and fig. 225 on the next page). Tapping the individual's hip or guiding the hip can also help.

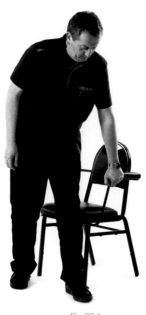

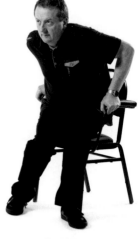

Fig 224   *Fig 225*

Beds

Lying to sitting on the edge of the bed is a major position change which will make some individuals so anxious that they just will not do it. Take the move in steps and reassure at each step. Rolling the individual on to his or her side first, drawing the knees up and then gradually coming up into a sitting position and then bringing the legs off the bed, can be easier to manage and produces less anxiety.

Rolling: thinking too hard about moving can create an inability to move, as movement is usually an automatic action to achieve a goal rather than a process we think about: distract conscious control by focusing the individual on an activity that would require a roll, rather than just instructing the individual to roll (e.g. stand at the side and say 'Can you look at my hand and reach or touch my hand?' rather than saying 'Roll over on to your side').

Releasing Grips

Consider the grip as a 'fish hook' (see fig. 229) **control the hand** (see fig. 227) **bring the individual's thumb gently towards his or her hand** (see fig. 226) **ensure the thumb is lying alongside the index finger and gently move the hand in the direction away from the 'hook'** (see fig. 228)

Stroking gently over the individual's knuckles may encourage the hand to release

OR

slide your hand under the individual's elbow and bring your hand **forward** until it is under his or her hand (see fig. 230)

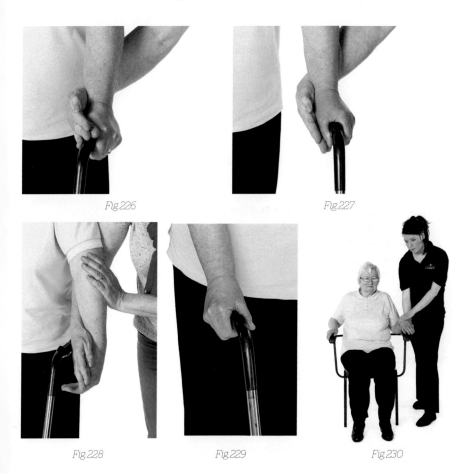

Fig. 226   Fig. 227

Fig. 228   Fig. 229   Fig. 230

Unit 20
Assisting the Plus Size Individual

Effective management of the plus-size individual requires a systems approach which encompasses policies, procedures, suitable resources, appropriate environments, training and a multi-disciplinary approach to risk assessment.

As individuals gain significant weight, their ability to move will be affected. Individuals put on body weight in different distributions and their shape can also affect how easily they can move. Plus-size individuals are at risk of airways restriction and shortness of breath and may need to sleep in a semi-reclined position.

The common body shapes are:

- **Proportional:** where the weight distribution is evenly distributed over the whole body and is proportional to height;
- **Apple:** where the weight distribution is evenly distributed around the individual's trunk;
- **Pear:** where the weight distribution is around the lower body.

Differences in body shape have an impact on ease of movement and how individuals move. Individuals may well have developed methods to enable them to move which suit their body shape and capability: for example, in getting into and out of bed, some prefer to get into and out from a prone position, while others will roll. A suitable, adjustable profile bed can be of great assistance both for getting into and out of bed.

Use of equipment to aid mobility becomes increasingly important for plus-size individuals in order to reduce the risks to the handlers. Even lifting legs into bed becomes a significantly hazardous task as not only may the weight of each leg be substantial, but also the individual's inability to bend at the waist will increase the effort needed from the handler.

Mechanical leg lifters are available or beds which are designed to convert from bed to chair to enable the individual to then stand.

Beds can also tilt laterally for position change and can often be made wider to accommodate the larger frame of the individual.

The safe working loads and the widths and depths of all equipment must be assessed, not just hoists and slings, but also beds, chairs, commodes, etc.

References

1 www.backcare.org.uk 2014

2 www.hse.gov.uk 2014

3 *Practitioner-client relationships and the prevention of abuse* (2002), Nursing and Midwifery Council.

4 *Management of health and safety at work – APPROVED CODE OF PRACTICE AND GUIDANCE, 2nd edition* (2000), HSE.

5 *Manual handling – GUIDANCE ON REGULATIONS, 3rd edition* (2004), HSE.

6 **Smith, J. et al,** *The Guide to the Handling of People, 5th and 6th editions* (2005 and 2011), BackCare.

7 **Oddy, R,** *Promoting mobility for people with dementia – A problem solving approach, 2nd edition* (2003), Alzheimer's Society.

8 **Muir, M and Rush,** *A, Moving and Handling of Plus Size People: An Illustrated Guide (Professional Series volume 3),* (2013), National Back Exchange.

Irish Legal System:

http://en.wikipedia.org/wiki/Law_of_the_Republic_of_Ireland

Terminology:

http://www.hsa.ie/eng/Publications_and_Forms/Publications/Safety_and_Health_Management/Workplace_Safety_and_Health_Management.pdf

http://www.hsa.ie/eng/Publications_and_Forms/Publications/Safety_and_Health_Management/Guide_to_SHWWA_2005.pdf

Safety Health & Welfare at Work Act 2005:

http://www.hsa.ie/eng/Publications_and_Forms/Publications/Safety_and_Health_Management/Guide_to_SHWWA_2005.pdf

http://www.hsa.ie/eng/Publications_and_Forms/Publications/Safety_and_Health_Management/Short_Guide_to_SHWWA_2005.pdf

Manual & Person Handling Training:

http://www.hsa.ie/eng/Publications_and_Forms/Publications/Occupational_Health/Manual%20Handling%20Revision%202.pdf

http://www.hsa.ie/eng/Publications_and_Forms/Publications/Occupational_Health/Caring_with_Minimal_Lifting.pdf

Safety Health and Welfare at Work (General Application) Regulations 2007 Chapter 4 of Part 2: Manual Handling of Loads:

http://www.hsa.ie/eng/Publications_and_Forms/Publications/Retail/Gen_Apps_Manual_Handling.pdf

http://www.besmart.ie/fs/doc/Manual_Handling_Health_Care.pdf

Safety Health and Welfare at Work (General Application) Regulations 2007 Chapter 2 of Part 2: Use of Work Equipment:

http://www.hsa.ie/eng/Publications_and_Forms/Publications/General_Application_Regulations/Work%20Equipment%20updated%20version.pdf

http://www.hsa.ie/eng/Publications_and_Forms/Publications/Information_Sheets/Patient_Hoist.pdf

Safety Health and Welfare at Work (General Application) Regulations 1993 Part X: Notification of Accidents and Dangerous Occurrence:

http://www.irishstatutebook.ie/1993/en/si/0044.html#zzsi44y1993a58

Notes

Notes